HERITAGE IN THE BODY

Global Change / Global Health
Janelle Baker, Cynthia T. Fowler, and Elizabeth Anne Olson

KRISTINA BAINES

HERITAGE IN THE BODY

Sensory Ecologies of Health Practice in Times of Change

THE UNIVERSITY OF
ARIZONA PRESS
TUCSON

The University of Arizona Press
www.uapress.arizona.edu

We respectfully acknowledge the University of Arizona is on the land and territories of Indigenous peoples. Today, Arizona is home to twenty-two federally recognized tribes, with Tucson being home to the O'odham and the Yaqui. Committed to diversity and inclusion, the University strives to build sustainable relationships with sovereign Native Nations and Indigenous communities through education offerings, partnerships, and community service.

© 2024 by The Arizona Board of Regents
All rights reserved. Published 2024

ISBN-13: 978-0-8165-5410-2 (hardcover)
ISBN-13: 978-0-8165-5409-6 (paperback)
ISBN-13: 978-0-8165-5411-9 (ebook)

Cover design by Leigh McDonald
Typeset by Leigh McDonald in Excelsior LT Std 10.5/14

Royalties received from the sale of this book will be donated to the Alejandro Pop Memorial Scholarship fund.

Publication of this book is made possible in part by the proceeds of a permanent endowment created with the assistance of a Challenge Grant from the National Endowment for the Humanities, a federal agency.

Library of Congress Cataloging-in-Publication Data
Names: Baines, Kristina, 1973– author.
Title: Heritage in the body : sensory ecologies of health practice in times of change / Kristina Baines.
Description: Tucson : University of Arizona Press, 2024. | Series: Global change / global health | Includes bibliographical references and index.
Identifiers: LCCN 2024005284 (print) | LCCN 2024005285 (ebook) | ISBN 9780816554102 (hardcover) | ISBN 9780816554096 (paperback) | ISBN 9780816554119 (ebook)
Subjects: LCSH: Mayas—Belize—Social life and customs. | Mayas—Health and hygiene—Belize. | Garifuna (Caribbean people)—Belize—Social life and customs. | Garifuna (Caribbean people)—Health and hygiene—Belize. | Traditional ecological knowledge—Belize. | Mayas—Medicine—Belize. | Garifuna (Caribbean people)—Medicine—Belize.
Classification: LCC F1435.3.S7 B355 2024 (print) | LCC F1435.3.S7 (ebook) | DDC 305.89597/9207282—dc23/eng/20240730
LC record available at https://lccn.loc.gov/2024005284
LC ebook record available at https://lccn.loc.gov/2024005285

Printed in the United States of America
♾ This paper meets the requirements of ANSI/NISO Z39.48-1992 (Permanence of Paper).

For Cooper

*Thank you for learning alongside me
in Belize, and everywhere*

I carry our heritage in my body now, always

It is a privilege to be your mama

July 11, 1999–March 17, 2024

And in my heart forever

CONTENTS

List of Illustrations — *ix*
Acknowledgments — *xi*

1. Change and the Body — 3
2. "I Will Go Back" — 27
3. "My Mom Don't Like Pills, That's Why She's Ninety-Six" — 49
4. "Your Money Will Kill You, One Time" — 69
5. "She Is My Doctor, She Dance Punta" — 93
6. Toward a Sensory Ecology of Therapeutics — 114

References — *139*
Index — *151*

ILLUSTRATIONS

FIGURES

1. Paving the road from the Southern Highway junction to the Guatemala border, Toledo, Belize — 4
2. Punta Gorda, Toledo, Belize — 24
3. The Split, Caye Caulker, Belize — 30
4. Thatch houses, Santa Cruz village, Toledo, Belize — 42
5. Marciana Alvarez at her home in Dangriga, Belize — 53
6. Mashing plantains for *hudut*. Bedford-Stuyvesant, Brooklyn, New York City — 59
7. Preparing caldo and tortillas on the fire hearth. Santa Cruz village, Toledo, Belize — 72
8. A young child watches the Deer Dance video. Santa Cruz village, Toledo, Belize — 88
9. Rosita Alvarez with recently harvested *cerasee* vine, Yurumein (St. Vincent) — 94
10. The Garifuna contingent from New York and Los Angeles boards the boat to Balliceaux, Yurumein (St. Vincent) — 98
11. Pig roasting for the birthday gathering, Santa Cruz village, Toledo, Belize — 123
12. (a) Maya Deer Dancer Basilio Teul, Santa Cruz, Toledo, Belize and (b) Garifuna Jankunu Dancer, New York City Hall — 135

MAP

1. Map of Belize, with key areas of interest — 2

ACKNOWLEDGMENTS

I WOULD LIKE TO EXPRESS immense gratitude to the Mopan and Q'eqchi' Maya communities of southern Belize and the Garifuna communities of Belize, New York City, Los Angeles, and St. Vincent. I hope I have told your stories in a way that honors all that you have taught me. Thank you for sharing them with me, and with the readers of this book. As I was told in Santa Cruz, "you have a lot of friends, Kristina," and I am so grateful to all of you and wish I could name everyone here. I am especially grateful for the loving memories of Marciana Cecilia Lauriano-Alvarez (March 1, 1922–July 12, 2022) and Alejandro Pop (August 18, 2001–April 19, 2021), one of whom lived a very long, full life and one of whom left us far too soon, both of whom taught me so much about the power of change and the useful plants of Belize. Many thanks to all my Belizean friends, with special thanks to Rosita Alvarez, Jose Mes, Hilda Mes, Basilio Teul, Gavino Teul, Anthony Cal, Amelia Cal, Hazel Arzu Martinez, Isaiah Sho, Elena Sho, Sonia Maas, Simiona Mes, Eluterio Mes, Ezekiel Canti, Lisa "Cookie" Carlos, Nickey Martinez, and Cheryl Norales. So many thanks to Cristina Coc, Pablo Miis, and Kaia and Imai Mis. Thank you to Filiberto Penados and Timeteo Mex. And always thanks to Francisca Bardalez and her family.

Thank you to series editors and friends, Cissy Fowler, Liz Olsen, and Janelle Baker for your inspiration and ongoing support. I appreciate you encouraging me to write through and about change. And thank you to Allyson Carter, Amanda Krause, and Alana Cecilia Enriquez at the University of Arizona Press for your swift work and kind advocacy.

Conversations with friends and colleagues helped shape my thinking and experiences around these ideas: many thanks to Becky Zarger, Anne Pyburn, Richard Leventhal, Josephine Biglin, Anne Pfister, Paul Kadetz, Sophie Haines, Lee Mcloughlin, Michelle Schmidt, Erik Stanley, Michael Harris, Alisse Waterston, Ron Loewe, Ian Harper, Judith Bovensiepen, Layla Hamadi, Hannah Graff, Denis Noble, karen g. williams, Maggie Dickinson, Alyshia Galvez, Molly Makris, Marianne Cairns, Alison Cantor, Aaron Hockman, Kerry Hawk Lessard, Kara Miller, Rick Wilk, Ria Banerjee, Jillian DeGezelle, Lyra Spang, Liliana Quiroa-Crowell, Angela Joseph, and Amy Thompson. Special thanks to Melissa Johnson and Jim Stinson for their generous and helpful comments. Thank you to Anahi Viladrich and my colleagues in the CUNY Faculty Fellow Publication Program for their valuable comments on the first two chapters of this book. CUNY also supported this work through the Book Completion award and two PSC-CUNY awards, as did the Institute for Citizens and Scholars with a 2019 fellowship. Thank you.

Thank you to my friends and colleagues at the University of Oxford who contributed to the development of the ideas in this book through countless conversations as I completed the draft: Elisabeth Hsu, Paola Esposito, Liz Hallam, Eben Kirksey, Laura Rival, Malvika Gupta, Stanley Uliajesk, Caroline Potter, Gwen Burnyeat, Anna Sehnalova, and Michelle Chew. Special thanks to the Pettigrew Family (Sally, Ali, Angus, Lewis, Olivia, Margot, and especially John) for welcoming me into their home for my final writing push. And thanks to the Baines family (Daniel, Lucy, Rosie, Reuben, Phoebe, Hobnob, Heidi, and Sparky) for getting me out of the library and into the cold river. Thank you to my oldest and dearest Cardiff friends—Natasha Bracken, Sarita Marshall, Arlo Taylor, Justin Kerrigan, and

Soraya John—for tapping into my embodied heritage with me. And thank you to Jeremy Hoffman for being part of these—and so many—adventures.

The deepest of thanks goes to Victoria Costa, the other in the "we" of many of the vignettes, particularly the more recent from Santa Cruz. Ethnography is life; thank you for sharing that with me these past twenty years. Please accept my boundless thanks for mothering alongside me with such care and intention, particularly through my many research absences. It is difficult to imagine the existence of any of this work without your ongoing support across every dimension, through all the changes, and I am fortunate not to have to.

HERITAGE IN THE BODY

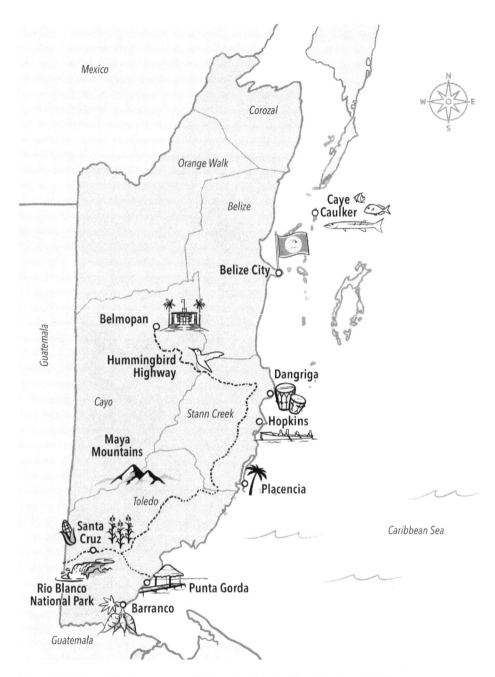

Map of Belize with key areas of interest. Created by Monique Boileau.

CHAPTER 1

CHANGE AND THE BODY

"I THINK YOU WILL MISS this place. You are used to it now."
"Yes. I will come back, though. We will see each other again."
"If we are still alive."
"Yes, if we are still alive."

As I left Belize a few days before Christmas in 2011, I could already sense the changes I would later notice when I made my way back over the next months and years. The rock-and-mud road I had struggled to negotiate for months had been passed over and made smooth in preparation for paving. As I got into my truck and drove away, waving and weeping through the village, the road became increasingly easy to navigate as I hit the stretch that the paving project had already reached, and then the stretch to the coast that had been paved for years. The members of the Maya community I had just left were speculating about what would happen when the road was finished, what changes it would bring to their lives, to their community. Would it be good? Would it be bad? Chances are, a middle-aged man said, it would be a "little bit good and a little bit bad." Whatever happened, they would handle it, they would adapt. As I drove swiftly through the East Indian community, which proudly announces its ethnicity on its roadside sign, I considered how a road might affect practices, particularly defined as "traditional" or related to heritage, that I had just spent the previous eleven months studying. As I soon reached the coast and turned to drive along it to the town, I noticed a small group of children playing in the

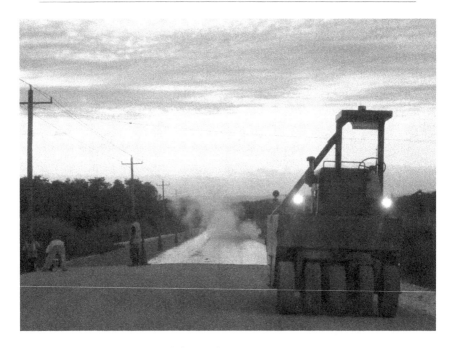

FIGURE 1 Paving the road from the Southern Highway junction to the Guatemala border, Toledo, Belize. Kristina Baines.

shallows of the Caribbean Sea. The nearby dock was showing visible signs of age, wooden planks askew, and a solitary fishing boat was tied nearby. I had come to learn some about Garifuna history and traditions from the little time I spent in town, and I knew things were changing here, too. While the road would make accessing natural resources in the interior Maya communities easier for those coming from outside, the resources in fishing areas frequented by Garifuna communities had been accessed by others for many years. Everyone felt the changes, past and present, and we all wondered what the future would hold.

CHANGE AS METHOD

Change is, in many ways, an obvious focus of anthropological inquiry. The process of leaving and returning to a community makes changes noteworthy. The cautionary desire for anthropological research not to become a simple snapshot, freezing communities in time, makes addressing change critical. The palpable acceleration of global environmental and economic changes gives the research urgency. I did not set out to study change when I returned to Belize the next year, and each year since, with the exception only of the 2020–2021 global pandemic. When I moved to New York City and reached out to the Belizean communities there, I was not aiming to look at change. But people feel change. They talk about change. And they live and practice through change. And, thus, change became a useful lens through which to see and begin to understand the stories and experiences of the Maya and Garifuna communities that shared so much time and space with me over the last decade. It became clear that lived experiences of health, of heritage practices, and of ecological systems and conditions, were better illuminated through, and impossible to disentangle from, a consideration of change.[1] And following this pathway emerging from and useful to communities reinforced the grounded approach to research I am committed to centering.

Following the changes has allowed me the opportunity to conduct research across time and space, focusing on the relationship building and relational accountability critical for community-based research, particularly in Indigenous communities.[2] As a non-Indigenous academic raised in a Eurocentric tradition, both personally and academically, developing these relationships was central. When I first came to know Belize, I taught Saturday

---

1. In my research, and throughout this book, I have broadly defined the term "health" to include aspects of physical, social, environmental, and community health. Using this definition, there is little distinction between health and wellness and well-being. I have chosen to use distinctions between health, wellness, and well-being only inasmuch as the participants in this research did so, and the distinctions were reflected in their own considerations of health. This health framework rejects the notion that health should and does refer to a more individually focused physical state and wellness, a more conceptual or intangible state.

2. For details on Indigenous research methods and research paradigms, see Wilson (2008) and Smith (1999).

classes in the Santa Cruz school building, excited to learn what the primarily Mopan Maya children told me about the local plants, and became a trusted teacher, before becoming a trusted researcher and friend.[3] As those children grew into adulthood, they shared their journeys with me and invited me back to meet their children. I was traveling back to Belize for the greater part of the last decade from New York City, where I had started to spend time getting to know the Belizean Garifuna community. My knowledge of Belize and Belizeans built quick trust and fast friendships in the United States that have solidified in that same decade and expanded back to the Garifuna community in Belize. These relationships made this book possible.

There are many ways to "do" anthropology, but most pathways share the basic desire to explore the microlevel outcomes of macrolevel processes. In other words, anthropologists are interested in how individuals, families, and communities consider and participate in social and cultural practices in the context of global forces. This study was driven by that generalized desire; however, the details and areas of focus grew from "ground up" ethnography. It was through ethnographic methods, spending time and getting to know Belizeans in Belize and in the United States, that my interview questions formed, and it was the answers to these questions that drew my attention to the macro processes that shaped them. There is no doubt that these macrolevel processes—for example, economic development, climate change, or political shifts—are worthy of investigation from multiple perspectives. Mine is firmly rooted in anthropological thinking and the belief that an ethnographic lens goes far in helping to avoid broad generalizations and deeply understand the experiences of individuals and communities. It is my hope that this book forefronts the human experience and makes the forces and changes impacting people around the world tangible through example. This tangibility is a strength of the holistic

---

3. For details of the educational program, please see Baines and Zarger (2012) and Baines and Zarger (2017).

anthropological perspective, illuminating the interplay between the social and the physical in context.

While the decade of traveling back to Belize to conduct research—and sometimes just to visit—frames this book, the primary ethnographic data were collected from 2016 to 2019, with follow-up in 2022–2023, and consist of forty-six semiformal interviews, five PAR workshops, thirty-four free lists and pile sorts, and hundreds of pages of field notes drawn from informal conversations and participant observation. I used a broad ethnographic approach, guided by both community priorities and my interest in health in ecological context. I took a primarily phenomenological approach to both the analysis and the storytelling, guided by the understanding that my own sensory experience as an ethnographic researcher should be clear to understand the observations I made and the thoughts and practices that community members shared with me. The result of this approach is this multisited, sensory ethnography that explores the aspects of daily life among Maya and Garifuna Belizeans that are broadly defined as therapeutic and occurring amid multiple dimensions of change.

"CHANGE IS GOOD"

Change is often assumed to be fundamentally positive. In many different contexts, people are encouraged to embrace change with open hearts and minds. There are numerous metaphors and clichés, such as "from cracked eggs come new life" and the like. Freshness and opportunity are all wrapped up into the idea that change is good for both individuals and communities. To return to the recent paving of the road in southern Belize as an example, this provided an opportunity for children to more easily attend high school in the nearby town, which, in turn, provided them with the opportunity to pursue work that required a high school education. This road paving is an example of how changes can be cast as a positive because they provide options. Infrastructure improvements—for example, roads, electricity, and water systems—are changes that allow for different daily practices, ostensibly saving time, extending possibilities, and even increasing well-being. This assumption is the core of the development ideology, which, although extensively critiqued by anthropologists, has substantial cultural underpinnings on a global scale.[4] Both the development assumption and the critique can lack nuance.[5] However, they are, in a sense, fundamental to the work of anthropology and anthropologists. Illuminating what communities define as "good" or "a good life" provides the foundation for understanding their practices around all facets of life: family, education, economy, health, migration, ecology, and more.[6]

The assumptions of the positive outcomes of a specific linear development model permeate not just popular thought but also existing governmental programs and nongovernmental organizations, which often encourage communities to adopt changes thought to be improvements to lives and livelihoods.[7] In 2012,

---

4. The development ideology referenced here has a long history of critique in the anthropological literature, notably from Escobar (1995), whose argument is that development processes have played, and continue to play, a strong role in the "cultural and social domination" of communities who are encouraged, primarily through globalizing forces in the form of governments and corporations based in the United States and Western Europe, to follow a Western-centric economic and social model of a "good life." For more recent discussion of development, see Nolan (2018), who provides a broad view of anthropology's role.

5. For a discussion of the how the anthropological critique of the tension between "seductive globalism and authentic localism" in the Belizean context contributes to a polarizing "drama" that has no clear solution and, in some cases, obscures the nuanced negotiations of daily life, see Wilk (1999). The stories in this book note this tension but hope to fill the space in between the poles.

6. For anthropological discussions of a "good life," see Fischer (2014) and, for a specific case study, Izquierdo (2005).

7. There is an expansive literature beyond that specifically promoting and critiquing development, from nineteenth-century philosophy to cur-

the year after I left Belize, I was invited to consult on a Belizean environmental NGO's project working with Maya farmers. Guided by the assumption that changes associated with economic development are intrinsically positive, the project enlisted me to investigate reasons why farmers may not be willing to change their land use practices in favor of allocating greater time, energy, and land to growing cacao for sale. From a development perspective, cacao is a more economically and environmentally sound choice than existing practices, and I sensed a certain level of frustration from project facilitators that farmers were not always compelled to action by arguments framed with this perspective. This change, to farmers, had both positive and negative elements, steeped in nuanced relationships between traditional farming practices and Maya values. Most striking was how the farmer's thoughts about making this change challenged notions of success and a successful life central to development thinking. Change is good, perhaps, if one's central objective is making more money. There are, of course, other ways to measure success. In this case, in Maya communities, growing corn to feed the family was a critically important measure of success or what might be called a "good life."[8] The social structures in place to support the planting, harvesting, and preparing of corn, coupled with the crop's centrality to defining Maya identity, are

---

rent popular psychology, which is based on assumptions of the primacy of thought and systems of living rooted in Eurocentric ideology. Specific critique of this literature is beyond the scope of this book; however, this volume in its entirety offers a challenge to it. "but also existing governmental programs": For a discussion of the role of nongovernmental organizations in promoting development assumptions and ideology, see Schuller (2009).

8. The disconnect and dissociation of those organizations providing capital for community projects from local realities and priorities is an example of how a top-down approach to community work is detrimental to community health. Understanding what it means to create "a good life" or *el buen vivir* in the context of global capitalist ideology is the subject of much scholarship (see Gómez-Barris [2017]).

livelihood considerations beyond just economics. This is an example of what a multilevel analysis, and deep ethnographic work, can contribute.

The "change is good" declaration is clearly evoked when family members encourage others to move location, often to places with the infrastructure in place to access additional options in the form of economic opportunities. However, all infrastructure improvements cannot be glossed as intrinsically positive. As a Garifuna man living in the United States told me about his relatives still living in Belize, with a tone of incredulity weighty with the "change is good" assumption, "I don't think they want to embrace change." He seemed disappointed that some family members in the Belizean coastal town where he grew up were satisfied with what he characterized as their cracked sidewalks and limited opportunities. Again, his notion of success was wrapped up in the ideology of development as change for the better. As a well-traveled professional who was grateful he had decided to embrace change, he felt strongly that it was, indeed, good for communities and individuals.

"CHANGE IS HARD"

Embracing change is often acknowledged as difficult, even if it is desired on some level or intellectualized as a "good thing." Again, clichés abound: people are "creatures of habit," "set in their ways," taking comfort in that which they know, frightened and resistant in the face of that which they do not. Anthropologists note the importance of ritual behaviors in human social organization as a way in which habitual practices can be understood.[9] Patterns of behavior repeated in specific, socially defined ways are ritual practices that provide comfort, and it can be upsetting when people are confronted with difference,

---

9. Anthropologists have historically used ritual practice in general and rites of passage in particular to analyze and underscore critical aspects of culture (for historical roots, see Van Gennep [1909] and Turner [1969]).

particularly if it is thrust upon them rather than presented as an option to be chosen. Many routine and ritualized behaviors become central to identity and group affiliation. Changing practices often means severing ties to place and to kin, both of which play such a central role in defining a person's sense of self and where or how one belongs. The stressors associated with these types of changes can lead to decreased wellness in ways that are easier to outline—such as increased access to processed foods or changing expectations of life stages—and those that are more nuanced, involving heritage practices and identity,[10] such as those discussed in the following chapters.

In southern Belize, Maya farmers often spoke about changing and unpredictable rainfall patterns making it difficult for them to schedule planting their fields, an important activity that requires several days of planning specific, prescribed activities.[11] The change in rainfall activity sets off a series of other changes, which have far-reaching consequences across society, the economy, and dimensions of individual and community health. Similarly, Garifuna fishers talked about unpredictability in the availability of fish leading to changes in social and familial structures. Both daily practices (for example fishing) and those that are seasonal and often accompanied by a series of ritual elements (for example planting corn) provide community members with a sense of wellness that goes beyond economic and food security. Maintaining them, for this and for other reasons explored in the forthcoming chapters, becomes increasingly important.

---

10. "such as increased access to food": For detailed studies on the effects of globalization and development on dietary changes, see Leatherman and Goodman's (2005) introduction to the "coca colonization" discussion with ethnographic research from the Yucatan peninsula and Cantor et al. (2018) for a more recent example from the Peruvian Andes; "or changing expectations": For a biocultural analysis of stress due to changes in cultural expectations and habits, see McDade (2002); "And those that are more nuanced": See Baines (2023) for examples in immigrant communities.

11. See Zarger and Baines (forthcoming).

"CHANGE IS GONNA COME"

Accepting the inevitability of change can be seen as equal parts ambivalence and pragmatism. Whether people like it or not, change happens, and they must prepare for the inevitable and roll with the punches. People negotiate changes in subtle ways, both preempting and responding to the changing conditions of their lives. It is this perspective that guided the decision-making of many of the Maya community members I have worked with, exemplified by the quote in the opening vignette about how the road was both good and bad and the next part of the assessment from the person who said it, a former alcalde: "Well, it's coming." There is an element of inevitability or personal powerlessness when it comes to individual experience of large-scale changes. That said, however, Belizean communities have been unusually successful in many ways when it comes to accepting seemingly inevitable development changes: notable examples include the public burning of genetically modified corn seed to avoid its introduction into the country and the failure of international fast-food chains to open successful branches in Belize.[12]

In the popular narrative, the effects of change on Indigenous communities can be oversimplified to evoke pictures of a cultural and physical genocide. There are certain truths to reckon with in this assessment; however, while the negative effects of climate change and global development processes on Indigenous and other marginalized groups are well-documented, so too are examples of resilience and adaptive practices among the

---

12. I have not sought data to substantiate the factors underlying the business decisions of the international fast-food chains; however, this discussion of the lack of these chains being at least in part due to local preference for Belizean food cooked in locally owned kitchens emerged as pervasive in my research. Other small, Caribbean countries with strong tourist economies do have many successful fast-food chains; however, a convergence of multiple factors is likely in explaining the outcome in Belize.

communities impacted by these changes.[13] It is my hope that this book will go some distance in illuminating this resilience without minimizing the real challenges these communities face, both in their histories and in their everyday lives.[14] Change need not necessarily be embraced or feared; it simply is a part of life, with moments of increased dimensions and intensities. Perhaps this moment, the "Anthropocene," as it has been termed in recent years, is one of these times of intensification.[15]

EMBODIED ECOLOGICAL HERITAGE

The effect of changes on individuals, of course, is more than a series of clichés, whatever truths they may contain. As I asked people about their health, I noted that answers increasingly

---

13. Zarger (2009) writes specifically about Belizean Maya adaptations to crises, in her case the global food crisis of 2006–8, and Crane (2010) develops the idea of "cultural resilience" as understanding how normative livelihoods interact with socioecological systems. These works challenge reductive understandings of the acceptance or devastation of development projects. Paranich (2018) continues this challenge in a discussion of cultural resilience in the face of climate change.

14. "Resilience" is a term some of the study communities here use to highlight their strength and capabilities in the face of adverse social and physical conditions. For a critique of the "resilience" frame used in marginalized communities, see Pugh (2014, 2021).

15. The "Anthropocene" is a term that has been used in recent years to define the current geological epoch. "Human activity is now global and is the dominant cause of most contemporary environmental change. The impacts of human activity will probably be observable in the geological stratigraphic record for millions of years into the future, which suggests that a new epoch has begun" (Lewis and Maslin 2015). Notably, anthropologists, particularly those working on environmental topics, have engaged with this frame as an analytical tool. The utility of its application has been challenged in recent years (see Todd [2015]; Moore [2016]; Latour [2017]).

included how changes across multiple dimensions—spatial, temporal, ecological—had manifested in individual bodies. People had moved for work, gone to college, changed their farming practices, and stopped drinking herbal medicines—for example—and they felt the impact of these changes in their bodies. With my ongoing ethnographic work guided by the embodied ecological heritage (EEH) framework, I have sought to capture how Indigenous Belizeans have navigated these ever-present environmental and economic changes throughout their lived experience.[16] Embodied ecological heritage kept my focus on the role of heritage, traditional ecological practices, and, more specifically, on how the individuals and communities I studied maintained healthy lives. People spoke about the maintenance and loss of "traditions" and of what it meant to be Maya or to be Garifuna in the context of changing practices. While heritage should not be conceptualized as a static concept, it brings with it a sense of continuity, in which the past informs individual and group identity, which was helpful to community members in the context of change.

I developed the EEH framework in 2011 during my first long research period, living in Santa Cruz, a small, primarily Mopan Maya village in southern Belize. The way that community members spoke about and conceptualized their health was intimately connected to how they spoke about "being Maya" or about participating in traditional ecological practices. The relationship between health and what the Maya community members defined as heritage practices existed on many levels and incorporated ideas about food, work, and education. The connections were simultaneously physical, mental, and social, with the healthy body described as that which could work and grow and prepare food in the traditional way. Their lived experience could be understood as EEH. This lens is useful describing health, particularly in communities that are not fully steeped in the legacy of Cartesian dualism. It is complementary to more politicized, critical health perspectives, which highlight structural forces and

---

16. Read more about the development of the EEH framework in Baines (2016a) and Baines (2018).

impacts on health.[17] Embodied ecological heritage is an important intervention in this perspective in that it allows individual sensory experience to be understood in the context of both the physical and the social, which is an aspect of health understanding that receives little attention. Bodies change through everyday practices, and these changes matter for health. Embodied ecological heritage guides the understanding and explanation of these changes, illuminating the role of heritage practices in the maintenance of health.

Embodied ecological heritage brings together seemingly disparate theories about the ways in which anthropologists have historically understood bodies and bodily practice. Phenomenology seeks to capture "being in the world"—the lived and embodied experience, felt through action or practice. This perspective has been set in contrast with more cognitive theoretical orientations, which aim to capture the internal structures of the mind and how they classify external factors they encounter. In my work, and through the development of EEH, I argue that these orientations need not be in opposition. Through a focus on how sensory experiences change the body (including the brain), EEH reveals how phenomenological and cognitive perspectives can coexist. Cognitive phenomenology as a theoretical orientation shows heritage is not static, not a list of traditional plants or foods, not simply knowledge stored in the brain; rather, it is something that is carried in the body. Embodied ecological heritage is a grounded theory: people speak about their heritage in terms of practice, or what they do with their bodies, and how those practices relate to how they feel. The language of sensory experiences—the smells, tastes, sounds, and feelings of doing and being in the world—is rich with connections to tradition, to heritage identity, to health. Documenting and understanding how these connections happen and how they form a critical way

---

17. Critical medical anthropology, as a theoretical frame notably articulated in the work of Singer and Baer (2018), emphasizes the macro political and economic forces that influence health behaviors and outcomes in communities. This analysis foregrounds the role of power in shaping health and illness.

of not only being well in, but also in thinking about, the world is vital.

BELIZEANS ON THE MOVE

If EEH demonstrates that there are links between traditional ecological practices and the maintenance of health, then how does change affect these links? If healthy bodies are those that embody traditional practices, it follows that maintaining those practices through change could also be part of maintaining health through change.

There are many dimensions of change, and they are oftentimes woven together. I focused first on spatial change, in the form of both migration within Belize and migration from Belize to the United States. Environmental changes, including climate changes, together with economic changes, often precipitated these moves, with individuals and families looking for alternative livelihoods in response to resource needs. While movement in response to change is just one of many strategies Belizean communities have historically implemented, it became forefronted in my research for two primary reasons. First, as the forthcoming vignettes illustrate, movement to and from Santa Cruz has increased in frequency and visibility since the time I began my field research fourteen years ago. Second, my academic position in New York City brought me into close proximity with Belizean im/migrant communities, which I began working with as much to connect with traditions and conversations (and eat food!) that had become so much a part of my own body after I had spent so much time in Belize as to develop a branch of my research trajectory closer to my new home, one which my undergraduate students could participate in.

Migration and the migrant experience have been widely studied in anthropology and beyond, as have the effects of migration on health.[18] Captivating transnational stories out-

---

18. For a detailed discussion on the relationship between migration and health, as well as a comprehensive bibliography, see Castañeda (2010

line lives lived through movement between two locations, highlighting links and divides within families and within individuals.[19] There is a nuanced layering of global and regional politics, neoliberal ideology, family dynamics, and cultural identity in descriptions and understandings of why and how migration happens. Anthropologists have unpacked and critiqued the trope of "in search of a better life" that infuses the popular narrative of what drives people to leave their homes.[20] The following chapters engage with this trope, and with these intersecting drivers, inasmuch as they provide critical context to understanding the stories told within them; however, the focus remains on the embodied experience of the individual. Again, I present this focus as a way of deepening understandings of maintaining health and living a good life, which might be initially illuminated by more macrolevel, political economic analyses—those same analyses that intersect with and critique the dominant narratives of development underpinning understandings of change.

The stories in this book ask and answer these questions: Is heritage practice therapeutic in times of change? Does practicing traditions, however one defines them, help in maintaining healthy lives? What role does sensory experience play in this increased wellness? In asking these questions, I am both expanding strict definitions of health, wellness, and well-being, and also explicitly investigating, through the lens of the EEH framework, how heritage is essentially carried in the body as it moves through time and place. Heritage becomes embodied through practice, often through practices that communities define as traditional and which researchers might classify as part of a body of traditional environmental knowledge or traditional ecological

---

and 2020) and Castañeda et al. (2015). For a more general discussion of migration theory in anthropology, see Brettell (2014).

19. For detailed accounts of negotiations of health and identity in a transnational context, see Gálvez (2018, 2019) and Levitt (2010).

20. For a detailed discussion and review of lifestyle migration factors, see Benson and Osbaldiston (2014) and Mancinelli (2021).

knowledge.[21] Examples of heritage practices encountered in my work include: preparing traditional meals, planting staple crops and herbs, collecting and processing wild plants and animals, making and/or using traditional processing tools and musical instruments, participating in traditional dances and music, and making and wearing traditional clothing. If participating in these activities is linked to wellness, then continuing these practices after people have moved is important for health maintenance among migrants and immigrant communities.

DECLINING HEALTH STATISTICS: IN BELIZE AND IN THE UNITED STATES

The relationship between health and heritage practices is a critical question to address given both the decline of migrant health over time in the United States and the concerns over increasing rates of chronic disease in Belize.[22] The healthcare opportunities and access provided in more urban areas can lead some to assume that health outcomes are improving in these areas. The statistics, as well as the anecdotal stories, suggest otherwise. If access to biomedical healthcare practitioners does not routinely increase positive health outcomes, it follows that considering health maintenance from a more holistic perspective is important.[23]

---

21. While often used interchangeably in relation to Indigenous knowledge and practice, the terms "environmental" and "ecological" have different yet overlapping meanings. While both refer to external surroundings and evoke ideas of nature or the natural world, "ecology" specifically refers to a relational approach to understanding the interaction between living things and their environments. This focus on relationships is an important part of understanding how health is maintained.

22. The rates of diabetes, obesity, and other chronic diseases are rising throughout the world. For an in-depth study of diabetes in Belize, see Moran-Thomas (2019).

23. For a more detailed overview challenging the role of increased healthcare access in reports of health, see Baines (2023).

The role of sociocultural factors in what has come to be known as the "immigrant paradox" has been both understudied and overgeneralized.[24] While the "change is good" assumption extends to migrant health, studies show, paradoxically, that change involved in moving from their home communities is often not good for migrant health. While less of an explicit paradox, this is also observed among those who move within Belize, with those moving away from their hometowns noting poorer health outcomes. The reasons for these poor health outcomes are often generalized across migrant and immigrant groups and include dietary changes (more processed, high-sugar, high-fat foods) and limited access to health services due to problems accessing a prohibitively complex system. Through using case studies developed through extended and ongoing ethnography, the following chapters go some distance toward illuminating how the lived experiences of those im/migrants interface with these biological and structural processes.[25]

"IT'S COOLER HERE. THERE IS A NICE BREEZE UP ON THE HILL."

I was sitting in a thatch house in Santa Cruz village in 2016 looking out of an open door down to the paved road below. Large trucks carrying cattle to the Guatemalan border passed by, as did small, white vans of tourists on their way to the waterfall at the national park, which had grown in popularity since the road

---

24. For a discussion of the "immigrant paradox" or the "healthy immigrant effect" specifically, see Hall and Cuellar (2016).

25. The research for this book was conducted as part of two main research studies documenting the relationship between traditional ecological practices and health, one in Belize and one in New York City and Los Angeles (IRB#s 2016–0249-GCC and 2018–0027-GCC). Funding for this research was provided by PSC CUNY, the CUNY Book Completion Award, the Community College Research Grant, the Guttman Foundation, and the WW Foundation (now the Institute for Citizens and Scholars).

was completed. There was even an occasional car, still a jarringly unfamiliar sight for me, as only trucks could have made it out this far just three years before. The wooden planks of the house still retained a fresh, reddish color, indicating the dwelling was not very old. I was sitting that day at a table and chairs and eating my generous lunch of rice and beans and stewed chicken with a fork, thoroughly enjoying it, but feeling uncomfortably like a tourist in a place that I had been invited to call home just a few years ago, when I would never have been offered a utensil to eat my food. While I was still much more comfortable having my conversations from a low stool and table, hands full of doughy freshly ground corn forming tortilla after tortilla, the conversation with the family of the house flowed freely that day. They had recently moved back to Santa Cruz village—the husband was raised there when he was young. They had chosen to come back and build a "traditional" thatch house after living and working for over ten years in a village to the northeast, along the highway and close to the capital city of Belmopan. They said it was because of the cool breeze that they had chosen to return and build their house on a hill at the end of the village. As their conversation continued, it became clear that the breeze was an indication of an easier life, a nicer life without the worry of finding money for rent or food.

It was not uncommon for young men and women to move out of the village to find work opportunities in this area, but people said it was getting a little more common to see people come back, especially people who were still considered young or middle-aged. Explanations for these returns often focused on an intertwining of economic and environmental factors, the forest, the river, and the breeze offering opportunities for traditional farming, harvesting, and processing activities. The subtle juggling of the opportunities of cash labor and traditional economic and environmental practices, which engaged with the land surrounding the village, seemed to be on everyone's mind. In 2007, Santa Cruz became one of two Maya villages in southern Belize to use the United Nations Declaration on the Rights of Indigenous Peoples (UNDRIP) to gain legal title to their customary lands. This ruling "officially" grants the community leaders their traditional rights to manage village land for collective use by all members of the village, allowing community members to maintain traditional farming and extraction practices, such as rotating cultivation and fallow periods, that would be rendered more difficult with the implementation of private land ownership.

While the sociopolitical implications of land ownership have played out in a different time frame in other Belizean communities, the narrative of the return to a cool breeze by the river is not unique to Santa Cruz. Sitting in a brightly painted Brooklyn apartment a few months later, I recorded a strikingly similar sentiment. A Garifuna woman spoke about her plans for the future, again weaving together environmental and economic concerns, as she relayed how a return to her home village meant a cool breeze, proximity to the river, and less worry and stress. In both the Maya and Garifuna examples, the connection between environmental practices and heritage traditions were made explicit and relayed through how those connections made their bodies feel.

I'M MAYA. I'M GARIFUNA. I'M BELIZEAN.

While the EEH framework can be used to explore, and even quantify, health/heritage links in any number of communities experiencing similar dimensions of change around the world, this book primarily focuses on two Indigenous communities with roots in central and southern Belize.[26] Apart from the practical reasons previously mentioned, these communities were chosen for their unique engagement with environmental and economic changes in the current moment. Both Maya and Garifuna communities identify and are classified as Indigenous groups in Belize (and in several of its neighboring countries), and they both have seats on the newly formed Belize National Indigenous Council (BENIC). There is a growing solidarity in

---

26. See Baines (2016b) for one example of how heritage/health connections might be assessed and quantified.

this indigeneity. Common experiences and histories are becoming more salient as sociopolitical events, such as the aforementioned Maya land rights case, which Garifuna communities have publicly supported. These events provoke a more pointed reexamination of the results of economic and social marginalization through access to environmental resources.

Coastal Garifuna communities have been impacted by changing land tenure policies, increasing in their intensity over the last twenty years as rising coastal tourist development and conservation policies effectively limit their access to traditional resources.[27] Maya communities have a more recent and visible engagement with the struggle to maintain livelihoods through control of their natural resources. There is overlap in these broad engagements, as well as in more subtle ways, such as the heightened focus on the importance of "ground food" and bananas/plantains to maintain a healthy diet. The formation and articulation of multiple identities, first as Maya or Garifuna, and, then, as Belizean, also provides areas of overlap, particularly in discussions of heritage and how that manifests.

There are, of course, many points of divergence. Maya and Garifuna people in Belize have very particular and very different histories, which predate the nation of Belize by hundreds and thousands of years.[28] These histories are told in this book

---

27. For more on the impact of tourism development on local Garifuna communities in Hopkins, see Appah (2018).

28. Maya people in Belize draw differing degrees of historical and heritage connections to the ancient Maya communities, which archaeologists have widely studied. The narrative of the "collapse" of the ancient Maya empires has a variable significance for the construction of identity among different individuals, some of whom express concern that the narrative erases the fact that the Maya are "still here." Garifuna people draw differing degrees of historical and heritage connections to West African people who gained freedom after the wreck of a slaving ship off the coast of St. Vincent and built their community with the Arawak and Carib Indigenous people living there. The narrative surrounding enslaved populations has a variable significance for the construction of Garifuna

inasmuch as they form part of the lived experience of the Maya and Garifuna people whose stories are written here. I am less interested in the "truth" of histories from the perspective of the colonial historians who wrote them than in how they inform how people define and practice their heritage. My aim is to further define how the ideas of what it means to be a good and healthy Maya person or Garifuna person or Belizean person are made manifest and carried in the body.

Belize is home to multiple ethnic groups, and, while there is a pan-Belizean sense of "One Belize" and many mixed families, ethnic identity remains central in much of communication and practice.[29] Kriol Belizeans have historically been seen as the dominant ethnic group and continue to hold many of the political and professional positions in Belize. While there is an acknowledgment that this is changing, Indigenous communities, particularly the Mopan and Q'eqchi' Maya in southern Belize, are still the subject of stigmatization, often related to their reliance on "the bush" for their livelihoods. As international recognition of the benefits of small-scale farming to nutritional health and overall well-being of societies increases, some of these stigmas are receding; however, they are still evident in the desires of some youth to distance themselves from these Indigenous practices and identities, particularly as engagement with formal schooling increases.

Belizean Maya and Garifuna communities' health conceptions and wellness practices, while not homogenous within or between groups, have considerable points of convergence. They share a holistic view of health promotion and maintenance, as well as of healing practice, which accounts for interactions with natural elements, ancestral spirits, and other organisms as experienced by the self and the family/community. In Belize, there is considerable overlap in the medicinal plants used and also in the foods classified as healthy. Trained practitioners outside of

---

identity among different individuals, many of whom critically emphasize that Garifuna people were never slaves.

29. For a discussion of the development of ethnic identity and its role in Belize today, see Cunin and Hoffman (2013).

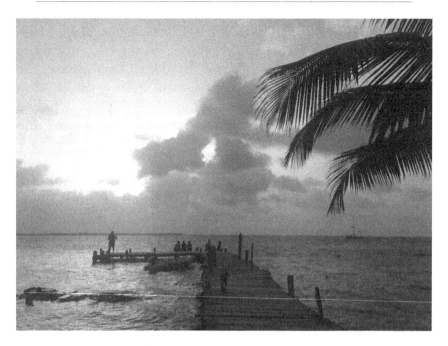

FIGURE 2 Punta Gorda, Toledo, Belize. Kristina Baines.

the biomedical system lead healing sessions, which combine the administration of medicinal herbs with other sensory engagements, such as singing or the burning of incense. Many of the practices associated with healing in the context of spirituality, most notably traditional music and prayer, are conducted in or adjacent to the Catholic Church, both in Belize and the United States. Both communities in Belize increasingly engage the biomedical system when time and/or money permits; however, as the following stories show, the health of the body among members of both Maya and Garifuna remains connected in a broad sense to the health of the community as well as the health of the environment.

CASE STUDIES

The chapters that follow trace individuals and their extended families through explorations of how health, identity, and heritage are conceptualized and practiced in the changing environments. The people featured here are moving through both space and time. Their stories illustrate how change, and responses to it, is sometimes marked but often subtle and how it can be noted in the body. Their stories of change are explicitly woven into their conceptions of heritage and what counts as a traditional practice. I did not pose any restrictions on the practices I was interested in learning more about; however, in working with the individuals and communities featured in this study, I was clear that I was not simply interested in what occurred at special cultural festivals and celebrations (although these were great fun and good opportunities to meet people). I was interested in the everyday experiences and embodiments of heritage.[30] I recognized the value of understanding the everyday practices throughout my fieldwork experiences and aimed to understand further how heritage practice is integrated into lives filled with work schedules, commutes, bureaucracy, and, in the case of New York City at least, the ubiquitous availability of slices of dollar pizza.

While migration and wage labor often come with an assumption of loss of traditional practice, this book pushes back against that assumption. It explores the opportunities new environments provide for an intensification of traditional practice. While fetishizing traditional practices for tourists is long discussed as problematic, the opportunities to engage in traditional practices and cash labor simultaneously opens possibilities. If migration and multidimensional change can spark an intensification of heritage practices rather than a loss—or at least in addition to a loss—the story of the Anthropocene might seem a little less grim. If heritage is understood as not static but as defined and redefined through change and practice, the notion of loss itself becomes overly finite and simplistic, and the notion of progress

---

30. Writing about Creole Belizeans in the context of movement and change, Johnson (2019, 145) notes that "quotidian modes of being, in backyards and kitchens, are powerful sites for the formation of cultural identities." I have found this to be the case in my interactions as well and am guided by these everyday experiences as best as I was able to capture them.

is redefined. Perhaps, like all good ethnographic volumes, this book aims to challenge notions of progress, opportunity, and success through confronting the lived realities of Indigenous Belizeans.

In a sense, this is everyone's story—one of adaptation, broadly defined, of building the best life amid changes largely out of our control. However, it is not really the story of transnational flows or development process, not really the story of migration or of climate disaster, although all these stories are worth telling in their own right—and they all intersect with this one. This is the story of the lived, sensory experience of individuals. This is a story of how heritage is defined, carried, replicated, and changed within the body through practice. This is the story of how our health is connected to that process.

As an anthropologist, I choose which stories to tell. This is, for better or worse, the seat of academic power—to illuminate, to contribute, and, perhaps still controversially, to affect change. Anthropologists experience and record so many stories and are trusted to select and to share in ways that represent communities and individuals in ways that they find true, important, and useful. These tenets may be self-evident, but they are forefronted in my process of writing this book. In selecting these stories, I am aware that there are hundreds of others I might have told—stories of heritage and embodied practice, of lives lived through changes, rich in social and environmental knowledge. It is my hope that the stories I have selected honor the diversity and richness of all those shared with me. It is my hope that these stories tell the truths of change, of progress, of struggle, of identity, of being and keeping well into the future. And it is my hope that, in them, the Maya and Garifuna people who so generously shared with me, and all the other potential readers of this book, find our common humanity.

CHAPTER 2

"I WILL GO BACK"

"**THIS IS A SPOT-FINNED BUTTERFLYFISH.** Spot. Finned. Butterfly. Fish."

And with those clearly spoken words, Isaiah popped his snorkel back in his mouth and dove down underneath the clear, blue water, a string of bubbles retracing his path back to the surface. We watched as he pointed to the butterflyfish and several other brightly colored reef fish hanging out under the coral ledges. He surfaced again, checked that everyone was doing okay, and led us over to the area of the reef with the swim-throughs. He had instructed me to take a photograph of him swimming through the rocky passage. I was to show it to his wife, Elena, when I reached Santa Cruz. We were in Caye Caulker, a favorite island destination for both Belizean and foreign tourists just a short ferry ride from Belize City. As I followed his bright blue swim shorts and dive skin shirt, snapping photos as his body floated gracefully in and out of the coral rock formations, I thought about what Elena might think of this underwater world her husband was inhabiting. It certainly would be a foreign place to her. I would later confirm my suspicions that she had never been to visit Isaiah here, never been in the ocean, never seen a coral head or a butterflyfish.

For me, this was a collision of my worlds. Having snorkeled since I was a child, and having learned to scuba dive while still a teenager, I was very familiar with the landscape Isaiah was guiding me through now, in 2018. I had also grown very familiar with the forest landscape of his home village, where his wife and children remained, and to which I would return and share the photos of his new underwater world. Considering these two places in tandem, connected through the swift kick of Isaiah's fins and my capturing of his image, I felt the changing construction of my own heritage and my own practice as an ethnographer, an environmental educator, a tourist, a friend. I wondered how such a collision of place and experience might be changing Isaiah's heritage practices—and how he and his family in southern Belize negotiated what seemed to me, in that moment, to be such a deep chasm of difference—of remarkable change.

A few weeks earlier, when I arrived back in Santa Cruz, I began my usual catching up after almost a year away. "What's new in Santa Cruz?" I asked, as I remarked on how much the children had grown, met the new babies, and recharged my body with bowls of much-missed caldo and fresh corn tortillas. "Nothing" was the usual response, but then the details of who had come back and who had left began to flow. It was when I asked about Isaiah's only son, Lester, who had been one of the top students in the Saturday classes I had taught for children in the village eight years previously, that I began to learn more details about his father's journey. There had been a steady increase of children attending high school after completing their primary school education in the village. While primary school was compulsory, high school was optional. And even though most parents supported their children if they desired to attend high school, there was a consistent acknowledgment of the difficulties the choice to attend posed to families in rural villages.

Previously, before the paving of the road, the daily journey to high school began before dawn as buses slowly navigated the rock-and-mud road, often taking well over an hour to reach their destination. The similar return journey meant that buses would often reach the village close to dusk, with children navigating household tasks and then homework by gas lamp or candlelight. Apart from the hardship of this journey for the individual students, families would have to do without the help of these older children for the entire day, putting a strain on many household-level daily tasks, such as meal preparation. The high school timeline also meant that students were unable to carry food for lunch because it had not yet been prepared when their journey began. This formed part of the financial strain on families, with students needing money to buy lunch—or going without food until they reached home in the evening if they did not have money. Stigma also played a role in food choice, with students stating that they felt self-conscious about bringing "Maya food" to school and wanting to eat "Belizean food" like their classmates. This tension between "Maya" and "Belizean" practices also played out in the preferred clothing and supplies students attending high school needed and desired in order to "fit in" among their counterparts from town or other villages, representing Belize's many ethnic identities.[1] Now that the road had been paved, and more families had access to solar-powered lights, the number of students attending high school was increasing.

While the easing of infrastructure and logistical pressures should not be underestimated in explaining the increase in high school attendance, explanations frequently indicated an internalization of the idea of "development as progress" described in the context of the "change is good" ideology in chapter 1. The global narrative assumes that increased participation in extended formal education increases a child's ability to succeed. Critiques of this narrative have been cautious, as it is difficult

---

1. Belize historically recognizes five main ethnic groups: Kriol, Maya (Mopan, Q'eqchi', Yucatec), Garifuna, East Indian, and Mestizo. There are also significant numbers of European-descended Mennonites and people identifying as ethnically Chinese. While there is a quickly growing number of blended families and those who identify with multiple ethnicities, food most commonly referred to as "Belizean" is most closely linked to Kriol cuisine.

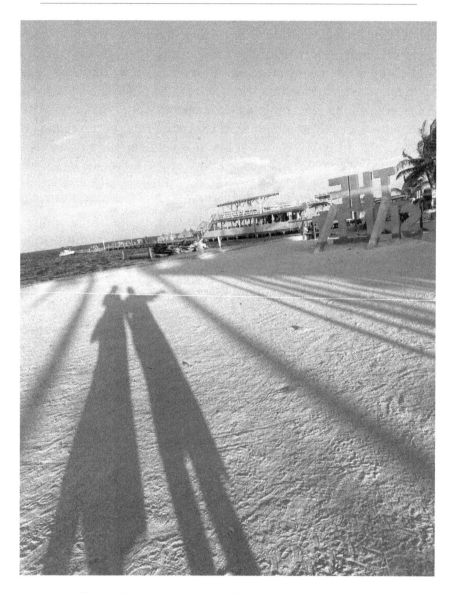

FIGURE 3 The Split, Caye Caulker, Belize. Kristina Baines.

to make an argument that a child should *not* be allowed to go to school and continue their education as desired. However, throughout my time in Santa Cruz, as supportive parents worked hard to provide these extended educational opportunities for their children, those same parents repeatedly offered a critique of this development in the form of many nuanced articulations and demonstrations. Elena was one such parent, as I found out during my next visit a few days later. Amid the graduations, the weddings, and the planting of corn, I witnessed ongoing changes in the way formal education was simultaneously embraced and critiqued through practice. Community members consistently highlighted the value of traditional ecological knowledge and practice, even in the families of the top students.

VILLAGE TO RESORT

Santa Cruz is a rural village situated in the lowland rainforest of the Toledo district in southern Belize. It is home to about 450 people, who identify primarily as Mopan Maya, with a small number identifying as Q'eqchi' or of mixed Maya ancestry. It is, primarily, a subsistence farming community, with the majority of families practicing shifting cultivation, also known as slash-and-burn agriculture. In this, one of the first two villages to win the legal rights to customary land tenure in a landmark case invoking the UNDRIP,[2] land is not privately owned and farmers rotate the plots they cultivate based on rules and preferences determined on the village level. Each man in the village will typically make a farm, or milpa, planting corn in May, when the plots are burned, and again in the dry season in October, when plots are not burned. There are no irrigation systems used in this part of Belize, and crop success is heavily rainfall and weather dependent. While cutting the "high bush" or old-growth forest, drying, burning, planting the cleared plot, and harvesting the crops are all the responsibility of a single farmer and his immediate family, the work is time-sensitive and impossible to accomplish alone. For this reason, a complex system of reciprocal labor

---

2. Subsequently, the remaining Maya villages were denied the land tenure claim and then vindicated by appeal in the Caribbean High Court of Justice. All the villages are currently, as of 2024, in the process of title claim and implementation of the court order.

is deployed and people "help each other," exchanging a day of their labor for a day returned back to them when needed. As more young men travel out of the village to attend high school and, after that, to work in the towns and resorts for cash to support their higher education, or that of their siblings, the labor system is becoming increasingly difficult to maintain. Middle-aged men seeking cash labor to support their children through high school put an additional strain on the system. The erosion of reciprocal labor, exemplified by cash payments, is often discussed as an erosion of the Maya way of life, of Maya identity, of Maya values.

Isaiah was certainly not the first person from a Maya community in southern Belize to travel to Caye Caulker for work. In some ways, his story is quite typical; however, in others, it is less so. For him, high school was never an option. His father made it clear that he would work at the farm, and he left school at fourteen to do just that. He had been smart, good at his studies, but questioning the decision of his father was not something he considered doing. He was a good farmer, he married, and he and his wife had four children. His home, next door to his brother's, is comfortable—a traditional thatch house used for a kitchen and a newer, more modern zinc roof and cement blockhouse for sleeping. As his children grew to high school age, Isaiah began taking jobs outside of the village. Soon, he decided to enroll in tour guide training.

"He does his training. Forty-two days. Nobody helped him." Elena was talking about her husband's decision to become a tour guide. It was a decision she supported, recognizing that it had involved a lot of studying and that the final exam was difficult, particularly for someone who had never been to high school. Learning the reef fish was always the hardest, I observed. For Maya people, the exam sections on the forest trees and plants and on ancient Maya sites were not difficult—they were learning about things that they grew up knowing. Ocean fish, however, were outside of the realm of daily experience for most members of Maya communities in southern Belize. Isaiah, though, had mastered them. Despite her playfully dismissive demeanor,

Elena seemed somewhat impressed: "I don't know. He just did that by himself," she laughed.

I, for my part, was truly impressed. In the eight years since I had been traveling to Belize for research visits and accompanying students, I had never been to Caye Caulker, a sleepy island village-turned tourist destination about an hour's ferry ride off the coast of Belize City. Traveling there now as part of my consideration of change in the Belizean Indigenous context, I met people I came to know well, who patiently taught me about the plants and animals of the forest, about the farm and the importance of working together and maintaining Maya heritage practices and values to live a happy, healthy life. And now they were teaching me about reef fish.

Anthony sipped on his cold soda and flashed his trademark smile, his eyes narrowing under the brim of his ubiquitous baseball cap.[3] We were sharing our first meal in Caye Caulker, having shared so many over the years prepared by his mother, Amelia, in Santa Cruz. He was one of the many young people I had taught in Saturday classes who had come to work here in their later teenage years. Some were saving money for college; others, like Anthony, wanted to earn enough to go back to their village and build a house and start a family. I was curious about both the idea that getting married and starting a family required cash—an idea that was, of course, very familiar to me in a US context—and about the desire to go back to his home village to participate in these activities in what he described to me as a traditional way. He was working in a resort development on the northern part of the island and had to ride a boat to meet me in the village for our meal. Most of the property owners at the resort were foreigners, and his easy demeanor and smile had

---

3. Anthony is part of Isaiah's kin network: Elena is his great-aunt. While they came to work on Caye Caulker at around the same time, it is common for family ties to bring people to work on the island. Isaiah's sister, Flora, was among the first people from Santa Cruz to move to Caye Caulker for work, and other family members have worked there at various points over the last decade.

made him fast friends there. When, at the end of the next year, he did actually return to his village and got married, he told me how one of these friends had offered him and his wife, Renisha, his luxury apartment at the resort for their honeymoon. She had really enjoyed that time, I later learned, although she missed her family too much to consider a permanent move. Over that first meal, Anthony seemed excited for future possibilities. He knew he would go home, but being here seemed a means to that end rather than an impediment to it.

Back on the boat with Isaiah, I sat close to the bow and talked with him as we were carried back to shore. Reeling from the day we had just spent with the turtles and sharks, I wondered if he was having as much trouble making sense of this world as I was—how must he think about it? He enjoyed his work, he said, although moving quickly from a day on the water to his evening job waiting tables was tiring. The boat trips were not guaranteed, though, and he needed to take advantage of the work when it was offered. He missed home but told me he made sure that he took the small peppers from the bush by his house in Santa Cruz to bring to the island—so his food could taste more like it did at home. He needed his peppers, but, when he talked about them, he referred to them as "our" peppers. As our conversation continued, it was clear that his use of "our" referred to not just his family but to a more collective Maya community. Losing the connection between what we eat and who we are is fundamentally problematic, and, as I heard that day, and on very many others, the disconnect cannot be sustained if people want to live healthy lives. It is not so much a preference for traditional foods but an imperative for health maintenance that goes beyond the freshness or the nutritional value of food: this longing expresses a more holistic health connection at the intersection of identity. This was captured as he concluded when we pulled into the dock, "When I go home, she has my caldo waiting for me. I need that."

Elena wrinkled her nose and shook her head. "I don't like it." She was talking about when Isaiah came for a visit and brought her lobster to eat. She was not used to eating it, she said, and it did not appeal to her on any level. I shared a little about how lobster had once been a food that poor people ate in the United States and now is considered a food for the rich. She nodded to indicate that she realized it was a nice gift, but that did not change the way she felt about it. I was not surprised by her reaction, because the few times I had shared unusual foods with friends in Santa Cruz, there had been little interest. The development of taste and preference as it relates to identity has been explored through food in Belize and beyond.[4] My conversations about health and heritage frequently evolved into discussions of how critical food—in this case, "our food" or "Maya food"—was to being a good Maya person. I was not surprised that Elena was not interested in lobster, a food so closely identified with coastal communities in Belize, but I was curious about how she was able to maintain her access to Maya foods, particularly corn, with Isaiah working away from the village.

Lester, her oldest child and only son, I learned, had stopped going to high school and now maintained the family farm, providing his mother and siblings with corn and other local foods. While I was grateful that the pressure was relieved from Elena, who no longer had to buy food because Isaiah was away and not preparing a farm, I felt a small twinge of sadness, fueled by my knowledge of Lester's superior academic skills coupled with my ingrained "development bias," that he was not going to graduate. Elena's assessment of this, however, clearly articulated what ten years of research had led me to understand as a well-supported truth: high school was not always the sure path to a good life.

"Now, what I see is when a child comes out of high school, [they do] the same work as the one that's never done the high school—the same job they go and do. So, it's best for them not to go and spend money for high school. That's why I say now,

---

4. Scholars have extensively explored how Belizean identity has strong links to Belizean cuisine (Wilk 1999, 2002, 2006; Spang 2019). For a review of studies on relationships between taste and preference in relation to food from an anthropological perspective, see Sutton (2010).

because [Isaiah] never went to high school [and] he found a job." With the financial burden of high school, and the added pressure of having to do without the contributions of high school–aged children to the family, many families just did not see the value if job prospects after high school were so limited. Elena was certainly not the only parent to question its value and purpose.

Elena, Isaiah, and their children may seem unique in that they simultaneously embrace and reject what I am referring to as "development values." However, their family livelihood practices were not as dichotomous as they might seem, and pragmatism is a noted feature of Maya communities in southern Belize, with subsistence farming and wage labor occurring concurrently and consecutively with increasing frequency. Research throughout the region and beyond has shown that development, both the ideology and the projects, introduced with little consideration for the culture and values of individual communities affected by the process, can be unhelpful at best and harmful at worst.[5] Elena and her family's practices show that there are nuanced negotiations of these processes—increases in formal education, wage labor, and nonlocal foods, for example—taking place every day. The centrality of Maya values and traditions to defining identity and being well is clear; however, there is more to the story than carrying local peppers on the seven-hour bus ride to one's job away from the village to understanding how this is lived and evidenced. Although the immediacy of a village pepper in the mouth providing an evocative embodied experience is something I know too well (evidenced by my exclaiming *pa'ap!* [hot!] in my best Mopan), I wondered what happens to the lived experience of identity when swimming down through a coral formation replaces planting corn. How was this embodied change situated within the wider sociopolitical context framing

---

5. For an overview of the anthropological critique of development projects, see Gow (2002). For more recent discussions, see Koster (2020), Neveling (2017), and Mosse (2013).

the defining of priorities and values related to land rights in southern Belize?[6]

TENSIONS AND BODIES: THE SANTA CRUZ THIRTEEN

"Today we're in this room, and we're talking about rights to land, but if tomorrow a cruise ship company comes and tells us we're hiring a few hundred people, we're not going to be here; we're going to be there because there's a need for employment, a need for cash." Pablo Miis was sitting in my Queens apartment in 2019 after a day of speaking at the United Nations Permanent Forum on Indigenous Issues. He was quoting Alfonso Cal, the former leader of the alcaldes in southern Belize, encapsulating the conflicting needs and desires related to traditional livelihoods (subsistence farming) and wage labor.[7] By all accounts, Miis is an activist and advocate for the inclusion of Indigenous voices in

---

6. "In a landmark decision given by the Caribbean Court of Justice in 2015, it was upheld that Maya customary land tenure exists in the Maya villages in the Toledo district and gives rise to collective and individual property rights within the meaning of sections 3(d) and 17 of the Belize Constitution. This means that village lands are owned collectively by the community and individual rights derive from this. Care must be taken to respect the collective rights of the community and individual property rights of each villager. To guarantee the collective rights of the community are protected, customary practices regarding village membership, residency requirements, and entrance fees must be respected" (from a booklet of MLA village and customary law and practices that was distributed by Maya leaders and then recalled).

7. The alcalde system is a much-studied historical system of village governance that predates more centralized governmental systems of elected officials. The Toledo Alcaldes Association, supported by the Maya Leaders Alliance and the Julian Cho Society, brings together alcaldes from all the Maya villages in southern Belize to discuss issues and support the traditional governance process.

government policy, and he currently sits, along with other Maya and Garifuna colleagues, on the newly formed BENIC. He works directly at this intersection of change, and, together with the spokesperson of the Toledo Alcaldes Association, Cristina Coc, challenges the standard economic development model, working with traditional community leadership to create a new Maya economic model, which forefronts concepts such as identity and reciprocity. This work is critical for the future of these Indigenous communities and perhaps goes some distance in serving as a model for Indigenous communities worldwide, who have been historically and consistently disenfranchised by the colonial logics of economic development models. While community members recognize the value of traditional land management and safeguarding the rights to land through the legal system, they also need to find ways to generate cash income. This negotiation forms the central tension exemplified by my conversation with Miis and this story about Isaiah and his family.

While Belize, unlike its close neighbors, is known more for its blue waters and jungle ruins than its mistreatment of Indigenous communities, recent events warrant a closer look at how these tensions and struggles have played out. In the wake of the Caribbean Court of Justice legal land rights ruling, Maya communities have been increasingly scrutinized and subject to varying levels of support from customary land tenure both from within and from outside the communities themselves. "Bad actors" attempted to win over support for privatizing Maya lands with promises of jobs, or "gifts" of coffee and sugar, or small sums of money. Outside influencers took advantage of even the smallest difference of opinion among community members. As of 2024, the government has yet to issue the title to the Maya communities for their lands, although the process of land demarcation for the issue of those titles is in progress. The communities in southern Belize have taken a multipronged approach to the land struggle: the legal approach, as well as a clear articulation of the relationship between the land, their way of life, and their health. The maintenance of healthy people and healthy communities is very clearly linked not just to resource access but also to the ability to continue livelihood practices explicitly connected to the land in southern Belize. And that land is not historically bought and sold; it is collectively cared for and managed by and for communities.

In 2015 Santa Cruz—and thirteen Maya bodies—became central to the converging story of Indigenous land struggles, government oversight, and public opinion. A community member sold a house to a Kriol man in Santa Cruz, in an unauthorized transaction without the customary permissions. The house was inside the boundary of the Uxbenká archaeological site and violated both village and national rules protecting the site. After months of letters and formal notifications of the violations, the newcomer was asked to attend the *fahina* gathering at the community center and explain his refusal to follow the rules. At the meeting, he became agitated and threatened violence, at which time he was restrained by the village police, who then requested backup from the nearby town. While restrained outside the community center, the man was photographed by a passerby and the photos were shared with the national press, along with a narrative that cast Maya community members as acting improperly toward the Kriol man. As the narrative grew in the kitchens and parks around Belize, local police mobilized in the middle of the night, arresting twelve men from Santa Cruz, many taken from their homes without shirts and shoes. The police also arrested Cristina Coc, the aforementioned Maya leader and activist who had been present at the fahina that day.

The case of the "Santa Cruz Thirteen," as they were dubbed after their arrest, soon became the subject of far-reaching public outcry. Isaiah, whose brother and nephews were among the thirteen arrested, became a YouTube sensation when he took off his own shirt and gave it to his brother as he was escorted to the courthouse later in the day. It was not until over a year later that the thirteen were finally acquitted, although the court of public opinion had made its ruling long before that. With little knowledge of the details of and reasons for traditional land management and the fahina system of collective labor, some painted Maya communities as exclusive, unfair, racist, and greedy. My role as an ethnographer, as you will read in the following chapter, became to help frame the incident, and its resultant injustices and stereotypes, in the historical, social, and political context of indigeneity in Belize, which is intimately connected to the control and use of land. Through my research, I have found that traditional land practices are critical to health and happiness, forming an important part of what we understand as "Maya heritage." Heritage, however, is not static, but rather embodied through everyday practices—and this incident illuminated the critical nature of understanding the relationship between these practices and community health and happiness.

HEALTH AND HAPPINESS: BLURRING DISTINCTIONS

Three years later, in 2018, another group of Santa Cruz's community members were sitting in that same community center. They had gathered in response to our call for participants in a "health and happiness" workshop.[8] Women and men of all ages self-selected and came together in smaller mixed gender and age groups to discuss ways and places in Santa Cruz that they connected to health and happiness, defined broadly. The four groups each chose a high school student to be in charge of writing their input on large sheets of paper. The first activity involved listing words associated with health and happiness. Through laughter and heated discussion, group members decided on broad categories for health (food, exercise, medicine, cleanliness) and for happiness (time with friends and family). As the participants were prompted to give examples and specifics, a pattern began to emerge. While many of the categories were consistent with more standard development goals, examples were much more place-specific and reflective of Maya traditions and values.

---

8. This workshop was conducted in conjunction with Tasreen Rahman, while she was an undergraduate student at CUNY Guttman as part of her participation in the CUNY Research Scholars Program (CRSP).

The "medicine" category included *sacate* (lemongrass, used for fever) and *yamor* (a bitter herb used for cleaning the blood).[9] The "food" group included *jippi jappa* (an edible palm), callaloo (amaranth), and caldo and tortillas.[10] The "good hygiene" group included a tidy, clean home—an important Maya value. "Enjoying gathering together as one" was prominent in the happiness category, reflecting both the Maya value of reciprocity, described in detail in the *Future We Dream* document written for and by Maya communities to explicitly articulate their vision for the future, and much recent scholarship on happiness, particularly in the postpandemic years.[11]

The blending of Maya values and traditions with those associated with a more Eurocentric worldview, such as brushing teeth and eating from the five food groups, throughout each of the workshop groups is more evidence of the everyday negotiations carried out by community members. The multiage groups with the high school scribes no doubt allowed for what was learned at school to come through in what was listed.

After the groups completed their lists, the participants drew maps marking where these activities related to health and happiness could be found in the community. Again, the maps exemplified a blending of both traditional and newer places. The recently appointed health post, a small building renovated to house traveling medical personnel, made it onto all the maps, reflecting a national push to provide biomedical care—vaccines, for example—especially to young children. The river and the farm also appeared on each map as places central to health and happiness. The community center was marked as central

---

9. *Yamor* is also known as *cerasee* or *sorosi* in Garifuna communities and is discussed in chapter 5.

10. Scientific names: yamor (cerasee) *Momordica Charantia*; lemongrass *Cymbopogon citratus*; jippi jappa *Sabal Mexicana* (Cyclanthaceae family); callaloo *Amaranthus viridis*.

11. For more on the relationship between positive social relations and positive mental health/happiness from a multidisciplinary perspective, see O'Donnell et al. (2022), Kim (2010), Greene (1972).

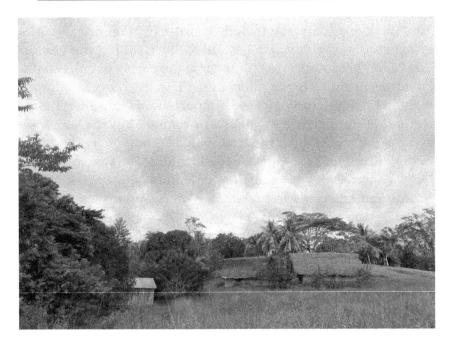

FIGURE 4 Thatch houses, Santa Cruz village, Toledo, Belize. Kristina Baines.

to happiness, reinforcing the importance of coming together for meetings and fahina. The centrality of churches to the maps captured both the old and the new: the Catholic church often being a hub for traditional music and other practices, and the Evangelical churches often being a hub for newer practices associated with their US counterparts (for example, playing guitar and keyboard through an amplifier).

While these workshop data warrant a more detailed analysis, the initial findings support and contextualize the role of both heritage and change in the way community members perceive and live their own health and happiness.[12] While cognitive classifications of foods, plants, and other substances have dominated previous studies of Maya health, recent work, including my own, focuses on how these classifications become far more fluid in practice. The lived experience of traditional ecological practices

---

12. See Baines and Rahman (forthcoming).

changes across time and space, and considering this experience is at the core of understanding health/heritage relationships. These data exemplify how cognitive phenomenology can be helpful as a tool to facilitate this understanding.[13]

RECHARGING IDENTITY

Questions emerged at the workshop about how such place-specific connections with health, happiness, and heritage—the farm, the community center, the river—could form part of the embodied experience when the body is so far away. In Caye Caulker, when Isaiah and Anthony both spoke of themselves, they spoke in the context of their families, their community, and their land. They both told me that they experienced their visits home every few months for caldo and tortillas as a reconnection of their individual bodies to the collective whole—an act both symbolically and tangibly connecting them back to the collective identity of "being a healthy Maya person." These moments of "recharge" acted as a buffer allowing them to retain health across seemingly insurmountable chasms of time and space. It is not surprising that caldo and corn tortillas are the foods of choice at birthdays, weddings, and other special celebrations—they have served a central role in many traditional ritual

---

13. My previous work (Baines 2016a, 2018) has sought to demonstrate through ethnographic account and the EEH framework that "cognitive phenomenology is not an oxymoron." In studies relating to environment and health in Maya communities, anthropologists have often relied on methods and analysis focused on the classification of natural substances (see Logan [1975]; Foster [1979]; Messer [1987]; Tedlock [1987]). These have been set in opposition to studies more oriented toward sensory experience as ways of understanding the natural world (Hsu 2007). Through a consideration of how bodies change through practice, the EEH framework demonstrates how sensory experiences intersect with fluid heritage conceptions, locating health and identity at this intersection.

practices. Interestingly, they are often still served at high school graduation parties—often alongside rice and beans and stewed chicken, the national dish of Belize. The negotiation of multiple identities is evident in what is on offer to eat.

"I will go back. I will go back in . . . actually I'm going back on my birthday!" Isaiah was sitting across from me, a thick, heavy wooden table between us. It was midafternoon, and we were at the restaurant where he worked nights, sitting under a thatch roof, cool on a hot summer's day. This roof was much larger than the cohune palm thatches back in Santa Cruz, though, and the thatch was made from bay leaf, or *xan*, a smaller palm traditionally used by Garifuna and other coastal communities and now often used to make the thatch roofs of restaurants and tiki bars that populate places such as Caye Caulker. We met up to talk a little more about his work here—and his family back home. I assured him that I did show Elena the photos of him free diving through the swim-through and that I had brought prints for him that day. He smiled as he looked at the photos—him pointing to an eel underwater, him feeding a pelican, him striking a pose on the bow of the boat. He slid them back to me across the table and asked if I would take them down to Santa Cruz and give them to Elena for safekeeping. His birthday was not until the following month, so I would make the journey down before he did. We chatted a little more about how his birthday is the day before my child's birthday, laughing at the connection, and he made a pitch about how I should come back to the restaurant for dinner because the fish, the lobster, everything was "fresh fresh." His salesman pitch felt strange to me in the same way that his reef fish identification did. I agreed I would return and asked him to tell me more about what was happening with Lester, who was taking care of the family farm back in the village.

"He's young. Yes, everybody say that. He's a young boy, but he still does a man's job. I think he had forty bags of corn; that's what he [harvested]. So, that's a lot." Lester was clearly an adept farmer, and I also knew him to be a bright scholar. The idea that high school would allow young men from the villages to be "more than just a farmer" was implicit in all the discussions about formal education I had over the many years, reflecting an assumption of shifting values around what constitutes a "good life" and perpetuating the idea that formal education and wage labor rank higher than subsistence farming in a linear model of lifeways. The many conversations that I have had in Belize over the past decade, both in and outside of Maya communities, have only lightly veiled the trope of the "backward Indian" or the internalization of the idea that one must excel in the colonial system of education to be seen as truly intelligent. This is not a particular revelation in development discourse or Indigenous scholarship, but on this breezy, summer afternoon, it was playing out in real time.[14] Isaiah recounted a conversation he had when Elena called to tell him that Lester did not want to attend school any longer.

"[I said], ask him, please, if he wants to go, because it's an opportunity for him. I don't want [that] one of these days, he will blame me. In my case, I'm a smart guy. I always came in first in my class. Ninety-six to ninety-eight is my average. And I did well on the national examination. I did eighty-eight. But my father was sick, and, in my days, we didn't have scholarships. So, that's the reason I didn't go. Thank God I can still survive. And that's what I told him. I don't want one of these days he blame me. I was gone for two weeks, then I talked to him personally. He said, 'No, Dad, I don't want to go.' And then his principal went to him two times about school and he said no. He said he wants to be a farmer. Everybody has their own hobbies, you know?"

I paused for a moment to think about the significance of Isaiah referring to farming as a "hobby." Was this his way of claiming a higher status now that he worked in the tourist industry? Farming would have almost always been considered simply work, something you need to do to provide food for the family, especially in the villages. While gardening or keeping a small farm in town could be characterized as something people did for fun, using the word "hobby" to describe farming practice in southern

---

14. For discussions on the historical valuation of indigenous knowledge and formal education, see Wilson (2005) and Dentzau (2019).

Belize stood out as unusual. This exchange demonstrated the complexity in understanding the tensions between work, both in and out of the village, and formal education. Isaiah and his family illuminate this convergence in unexpected ways.

CHANGES UPON CHANGES

When Anthony and Isaiah met me at the ferry dock in Caye Caulker in 2022 for the first time since the COVID-19 pandemic closed borders to Belize, there were some new changes to discover. As we drove around the island in Isaiah's new golf cart taxi, work that Isaiah had taken up to supplement the still-recovering snorkel guiding opportunities, they caught me up on happenings back in Santa Cruz. The football team was doing really well. Anthony's first child was eating well and growing quickly. People were leaving their jobs at the banana farm because more lucrative postpandemic opportunities were starting to return. I asked about Lester and how the farm was doing, and Isaiah told me that Lester was there in Caye Caulker living with him for a while and working at a local grocery store. Grateful for the warm wind blowing on my face in the midday July sun as the cart zipped through the narrow streets, I nodded, slightly surprised. "Do you want to go see him?" Isaiah asked, and I nodded again. The cart pulled up outside the grocery store and Anthony and I jumped off, Isaiah darting off to take an opportunity for a fare. Lester appeared and explained that he was not yet sure how long he would stay or if he might prefer to return to his village and farm again. He missed it, he said, and he missed his mom, but he was hoping to make a little money to make things easier for everyone. As he slipped back inside to work, Anthony and I walked through the narrow streets to a sea-blown wooden boardwalk, where we shared another meal, this time with watermelon juice.

"It's not a good idea to leave farming completely," Anthony explained. He was discussing his decision to return to work on the island after several years at home during the pandemic.

Working out of the village elicited more consideration and consequences now that he was married and supporting a child. He clearly missed them but had an explanation for how he could maintain what he considered important aspects of his traditions and "work out" [of the village] at the resort. He explained how he paid someone to take care of his farm—often a family member who did not have the qualifications to land a job outside of the village. That way, he explained, he didn't have to worry about not having enough corn for tortillas or for *poch* (corn masa steamed in a *waha* leaf, often served at large gatherings) when he needed them. It was cheaper to pay family and friends than to buy corn, and he was essentially spreading the wealth. It did not surprise me that having his own farm, particularly for corn, was important to him; however, I was interested in how he chose to frame the hiring of family members as supporting a value that he held as critically important: working together.

"These are the good parts that I see." We had finished our juice and were digging into a whole snapper. I was concerned that the fish was not big enough, but Anthony assured me that he was getting used to not eating a lot, because he had been spending so much time with tourists, who sometimes eat a few pieces of fruit in the morning and call it breakfast. "The good part is that maybe you want to go out to work and your brother wants to stay in [the village]. You work together and you get a little money and they get a little money and you still have your corn." Working together and having your own corn assures that you do not have to worry, he explained. Your family will always have what they need. "I call her every day," Anthony said of Renisha, his smile returning at the thought of her. He had moved his house—it was now very close to the creek and on a hill, so sometimes there is cell service there. He made a point of telling me that, although he liked the previous zinc-and-concrete house he had built when he first started working and before he got married, he was happy to be back in a thatch house. "We always prefer a thatch house. It's cooler; you can relax. And it's important to be close to the river." I nodded knowingly, having both heard these assessments many times and experienced them with my own body. As we finished our meal and looked out into the island sunset, I considered how Anthony's work involves helping others find their relaxing island experience, while he waits to go home and find his own relaxation under the leaves of the cohune palm, just as his ancestors had for hundreds of years.

CHAPTER 3

"MY MOM DON'T LIKE PILLS, THAT'S WHY SHE'S NINETY-SIX"

"I BEST NOT GO THERE; they're gonna tie me up." It was 2015 in the village of Hopkins, and I was sitting in a restaurant and bar, with smooth concrete floor and no walls so the sea breeze flowed freely, even though we were a couple blocks in from the beach. Those spots on the shore were now reserved for the new resorts and tourists looking to experience the idyllic Caribbean shoreline. My friend, another anthropologist from the United States, had met me at the restaurant, introducing me to her two friends—one Garifuna man and one Kriol man. They had grown up in this place—once a small fishing village and now a growing resort town—and had seen the changes firsthand. As we got to know each other, they came to learn that I had spent a lot of time in Santa Cruz. While it was unlikely they would have heard of this small Maya village hours away in the south just the year before, now the mention of its name sparked a groan, accompanied by a comment about being afraid to go there. Santa Cruz had been in the news and now people were talking about it.

As we sat together, sipping slowly on Belikins in the sticky breeze, I listened as my new friends relayed what they had seen on the news—a Black man on the ground, his hands tied, Maya men holding machetes. I then relayed what I had come to know as the truth of those images—that they had been taken during a fahina after the man had threatened the villagers with violence. He had moved into the village the year before, violating multiple aspects of village protocol, including damaging the local ancient Maya site. The village leadership, following established rules, had attempted to require him to comply, and when he threatened violence, the village police were instructed to restrain him and await backup from the police in Punta Gorda. This is when the images were taken—a misunderstanding at best, an intentional misrepresentation at worst.

The men considered my words, which told a different version of the story than they had seen on the news. They shared with me that they had heard that the man the villagers restrained had behaved poorly before—in his home village—and it made sense that he had been in the wrong. The conversation then took a deeper turn into the shared histories of different communities in Belize. The inhabitants of Santa Cruz had recently won the rights to their land, but the government was, and still is, in the process of implementing those rights. Land had been parceled and privatized in their village many years before, disenfranchising many of the community members. As the evening progressed and the breeze cooled, my new friends identified many more similarities with their Maya counterparts in the south, whom they had feared at the beginning of our conversation—similarities born out of these shared histories and shared ecologies, including relationships with governments and bureaucracies, but, first, with the land and the water.

FISHERS TO TEACHERS TO HERBALISTS

Hopkins is a Garifuna village, settled by Garifuna fishermen back before folks remember. Garifuna Settlement Day, celebrated on November 19 in Belize and by Belizean Garifuna throughout the diaspora and commemorating the arrival of the Garifuna people in Belize on that day in 1802, honors the resilience and longevity of what it means to be Garifuna—and how place plays a role in that meaning. The forcible ouster of the Garifuna from St. Vincent as part of the European-led Caribbean colonial genocide sent them on a remarkable (in all the senses of the word) journey, which scattered them throughout the coastal communities of Central America that became their home and, later, in substantial, thriving diasporas in the United States, most notably in New York City and Los Angeles. Tensions between coastal Garifuna communities in Belize and the historically dominant Kriol communities have, in some important ways, been mirrored by Maya communities in Belize.[1] The trope of the "underdeveloped" or "uneducated" fisherman, living close to the land in a kind of day-to-day existence, was contrasted with the formality of the British colonial government and commerce of natural resource extraction. Decades ago, Garifuna communities began identifying individuals who would begin a long lineage of excelling in school and training to be teachers.[2] Garifuna teachers were often given the most challenging or least desirable postings and sent into the most rural communities to staff schools deep in the forests, where they developed intimate and trusted relationships with the Maya families living there.[3] As these teachers developed seniority, they were posted to schools in Belize City or the other

---

1. Kriol or Creole, meaning "mixed" in Belize, refers to both an ethnicity and a language. Kriol communities in Belize trace their histories to British logwood and mahogany cutters and traders and their enslaved West African workers. They have historically been more likely to hold positions of power in government, municipal systems, and so forth, but this power has been actively shifting in recent decades.

2. Maya communities have more recently participated in identifying those excelling in school to train to be teachers. In part because of this process, which not everyone took part in, there remains a capital/class divide among various ethnicities, in addition to among Garifuna communities, in Belize.

3. For a detailed account of the lives of early Garifuna teachers and the hardships they faced in establishing schools in remote villages in Belize, see Enriquez's (2017) account of his grandparents' experiences.

more populated areas—and their children saw the opportunity to move, often with the family profession, to the United States.

"My mother don't like pills, that's why she's ninety-six." I was sitting in a comfortable leather recliner in the living room of a well-appointed home in the Bedford-Stuyvesant neighborhood of Brooklyn, New York City. Rosita Alvarez was talking about her mother, Marciana, who lived until very recently in Dangriga, a larger, coastal town just to the north of Hopkins in the Stann Creek district of Belize. She spoke about the traditional medicinal practices she learned from her mother, many of which she uses in Brooklyn, where biomedicine is the norm. Rosita leads a cultural group centered around the local Catholic church and is dedicated to promoting both pan-Garifuna and pan-Belizean identity and culture. It is a central part of her life and brings her much joy, as well as a certain amount of frustration.

"It's not easy. A lot of people who have come to the States are more into the American way of life. I do understand why because this is where they live. Everybody won't adapt the way they do. Some of us remain here. We live here. This is a Garifuna house. We live here, we speak Garifuna. But others, maybe they can't. Maybe they're not interested." This is a tension that Rosita and I have revisited over time as our relationship has deepened. In this conversation, one of many in which she has outlined the many ways being Garifuna is linked to leading a good, healthy life, she explained how she and the members of the New York City Garifuna community access the botanical materials, natural herbs and roots used in medicinal teas and topical preparations, in the urban metropolis. She signaled to me to wait in my comfortable seat and went to the pantry to retrieve a plastic bag. She opened it to reveal a pile of reddish-brown roots brought from Belize. When prepared, they comprise a medicinal brew used to cleanse the blood. The community, she explained, shares information about which Korean stores in the neighborhood carry the herbs that they would normally grow and harvest in Belize. Rosita buys lemongrass from the store right by her subway entrance. Ginger, allspice, and cinnamon are also purchased and used to maintain the health of bodily systems. I remarked that I had learned a lot about how plants in Belize are used in everyday medicinals from the Maya communities: lemongrass for a cough and a fever, allspice leaves for weddings and special ceremonies, bitter vines and roots for cleansing blood. She nodded, signaling that these practices were well known among other communities. Maintaining Garifuna identity through traditional practices, both in Belize and in Brooklyn, meant valuing how other traditional communities shared and maintained knowledge. In the context of the fears and cautions of a homogenizing, globalizing world, we shared a quiet acknowledgment that it is not just international pharmaceutical and technology companies driving cultural practice—she and other Indigenous leaders and community members are driving it with their bodies in everyday practice.

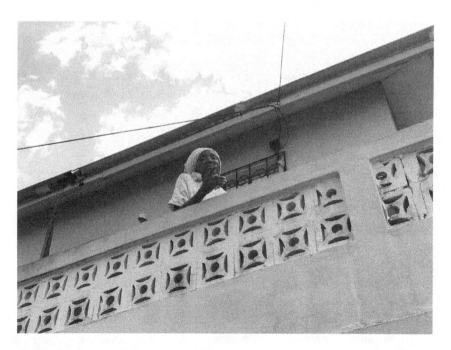

FIGURE 5 Marciana Alvarez at her home in Dangriga, Belize. Kristina Baines.

THE GREEN HOUSE BY THE WATER TANK

"The Chinese—they love it. They know what's good." A young Garifuna father, with thick dreadlocks tied neatly at his neck, held a small, green spray of leaves for me to observe. He explained that Garifuna communities here in Dangriga used to use this plant, but many people now prefer to get their medicines at the shop. The more recent Chinese immigrants and Belizeans of Chinese ethnicity—the most rapidly growing segment of the Belizean population—have taken to growing medicinal herbs in their front yards and this, he told me, is contributing to a resurgence in interest from the Garifuna youth in the community. He explained that the plant, Chanka pedra (*Phyllanthus niruri*), could be used to address so many of the health issues facing this coastal Belizean town, notably kidney stones and diabetes, which have been increasing at a frightening rapid rate, particularly among the Garifuna.[4] There was an urgency behind his coastal Caribbean demeanor—a palpable understanding that the youth of his community needed to hang onto, or relearn, their traditional plant knowledge to ensure future wellness.

This conversation took place in Dangriga, in the living room of the "green house behind the white house by the water tank," a house that belonged to Rosita's mother, Marciana, which I found using directions given to me back in Brooklyn. The young father giving this botanical lesson was the taxi driver (known locally as "Heads"), who had known the house and brought us here from the bus station. He was related to the family as a cousin. When we called upstairs for Ms. Alvarez, Marciana appeared from the elevated mint-green building and looked out over the white stone rail of the porch, her ninety-six-year-old eyes slowly focusing on the unexpected visitors below. We announced ourselves as Rosita's friends from New York and

---

4. In her detailed account of diabetes among Garifuna communities in Belize, Moran-Thomas (2019) documents the disproportionate and alarming rates of diabetes among Garifuna communities in Belize.

were quickly invited in for a visit. I asked her the secret to her good health and longevity and mentioned that Rosita had told me about how she "don't like pills." She agreed and then took us on a tour of the plants growing around her house. We stopped at each one: mango, prickly pear cactus, more, and she explained how each had helped to keep her well.[5] When we returned to the living room, she asked me to encourage her grandchildren in Brooklyn to write to her more often and then challenged Heads to explain what plants he used, prompting the discussion detailed above.

Leaving Marciana's home more quickly than I wanted to catch the next bus, I considered the role of time in the practice of being well. In one sense, it felt jarring to my body to leave her home so quickly in that moment, which had easily slipped back into the rhythm of Belize, where slow visits are the norm. However, my body had spent many years growing more accustomed to the pace of life in New York City, of moving quickly to the next appointment or activity. Living and learning through both locations had begun to teach me not just about the spatial dimension of change but also about the temporal dimension in which speed is captured through embodied practice: the stretching to match the growth of the mango tree, the waiting for a letter to be delivered and then holding it in your hand, the processing of roots and herbs. It seems obvious to observe the temporal nature of heritage practices, which by definition are linked to the past. Through an expansive definition of heritage, however, the fluidity of tradition, which can be lost in spaces like Dangriga town, may be reimagined through practice in Brooklyn and then surface in new embodiments over time, through the Chinese Belizean community in this example. The body recalls and enacts across the changes of time and space.

---

5. For more on the importance of kitchen gardens from a health perspective, see Mundel and Chapman (2010) and Finerman and Sackett (2003).

PROGRESS: TALES FROM THE SIDEWALK

Several months later, I was back in Brooklyn sitting on Rosita's stoop chatting to her son-in-law about his choice to leave Belize and build his life in the United States. We were looking out at the sidewalk in front of us as he explained what he meant when he talked about a lack of motivation and resources for development in his hometown in Belize. He noted the cracks in the pavement—in Belize, they don't get fixed. As someone who is consistently interrogating what it is, people—scholars, community members, organizations—actually mean when they talk about "development," this seemed like a pretty concrete example, pardon the pun. The lack of attention to infrastructure maintenance was a clear example, to him, of a certain attitude he noted in Belize—one that factored into his decision to leave. Repairing sidewalks was not a priority for his Garifuna community in Dangriga. As the conversation developed, and again included Rosita and other family members, it became clear that teasing out what really defined progress was not as easy as cracks in the concrete, however compelling the simplicity of both the example and the metaphor, which became even more captivating after I learned that *Chanka piedra* (the "stone breaker") was noted for growing in cracks in the pavement. I asked if living in the United States was generally better in terms of progress.

"Well, I guess, for the opportunities, it is. It's a trade-off—[there is] more opportunity as far as jobs, but as far as freedom and safety, [it's better in Belize]." I considered what the juxtaposition of freedom and safety meant in the wider context of Indigenous identity and health. These terms were, to me, very much steeped in an American notion of progress, as it relates to an assumption of desire. People come to the United States to experience freedom and safety in the form of economic opportunities yet sometimes encounter violence. In this conversation, the increase in job opportunities, which could be considered an aspect of freedom to some, is set in opposition to it. Through this conversation, and many others like it, the notion of freedom has come to capture aspects of life and perspective that change through the assimilation and acculturation processes, processes once thought to be necessary to live a healthy, fulfilled life in the receiving country.[6] The freedom to retain certain traditions, to live close to the land if you choose, to live outside of certain bureaucratic structures—these are the freedoms that are lost with acculturation. Looking solely to acculturation models to explain immigrant health has been widely critiqued, with the critics' main points focusing on structural rather than cultural barriers to health.[7] A consideration of structural racism and intersectionality through the lens of immigrant health allows for a deeper consideration of why freedom and safety seem more accessible in Belize. Garifuna identity encompasses both Indigenous and West African traditions; however, the nuances of this identity are not manifested in the same way across the everyday experiences of race and racialization across the diaspora.

While Rosita's Brooklyn neighborhood is a historically Black American community, it is also surrounded, like much of New York City, by many other Afro-Caribbean communities that distinguish themselves from Black Americans through traditional practices.[8] This distinction is not as salient in the negotiation of everyday life in US cities, where race and racism are active considerations of living life in a black-and-brown body. Perhaps this is where a deeper consideration of safety comes into play. As noted before, it is not as if racial and ethnic marginalization do

---

6. Outdated and nationalist approaches often encouraged immigrants to assimilate into their receiving country. This approach is perhaps most familiar in the once-popular trope "You're in America now!"

7. In Viruell-Fuentes et al. (2012), structural racism and intersectionality theory are proposed as a more complete analysis of immigrant health, challenging outdated models of acculturation as useful approaches for understandings or recommendations supporting immigrant health.

8. There is much literature detailing the lives and traditional practices of Afro-Caribbean communities in New York City. For a discussion of traditional foodways in the substantial Dominican communities, see Fuster and González (2019). For a detailed discussion of these practices in the Honduran Garifuna community, see England (2023).

not exist in Belize—they do—but navigating these is easier there because they are less stark and Blackness is not minoritized. The threats to freedom and safety in Belize, for Garifuna people, are less embedded, less ever-present.

"It's part of our DNA!" We moved from the sidewalk to the dinner table. Rosita had made *hudut*, a traditional Garifuna soup of fresh fish, herbs, mashed plantains, and coconut milk, and the family was eagerly awaiting its arrival on the table. I asked why they are so excited to eat it; why, after all these years living and working in the United States, they still love it so much. It is clear that my question was almost ridiculous to them—and ridiculous beyond the fact that hudut is so very delicious. If you are Garifuna, eating hudut is part of who you are. It is in your DNA. Identity fundamentally sits at the intersection of the biological and the social. This recognition of this convergence, perhaps, has never been more at the forefront of popular thought than it is now. The advent of the home DNA testing kit has played a substantial role in thinking about what it means to be 30 percent Ghanan or 60 percent German or, perhaps most controversially, part Indigenous. In a comical nod to, and erasure of, cultural identity, the television advertisements for the kits flash from someone dressed in lederhosen that magically disappear when they find out they are not in fact German, as if finding out the details of one's DNA will instantly change one's cultural practices. As cultural anthropologists, we are acutely attuned to how much of behavior is mitigated by culture and are often embroiled in a near constant fight against those who offer a fixed, and often genetic, analysis of behavior. This latter view, in my experience, permeates popular imagination and is likely one of the roots of the popularity of these tests. Understanding your genes, it is thought, enables you to understand who you are.[9]

The popularity of finding out who you are, in this context, demonstrates how the importance of heritage practices has been internalized; it also shows concerns over the loss of those

---

9. For a discussion of DNA testing and ancestry from an anthropological perspective, see Shelton and Marks (2001) and Abel and Frieman (2023), with a broader discussion found in Marks (2013).

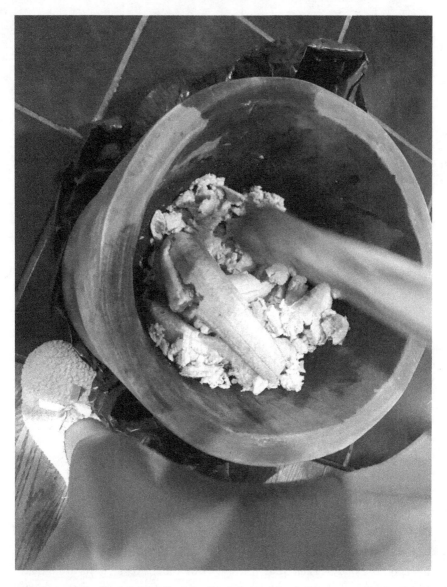

FIGURE 6 Mashing plantains for hudut. Bedford-Stuyvesant, Brooklyn, New York City. Kristina Baines.

practices being passed down through the generations. If the practices and rituals associated with heritage are related to health, accessing and engaging in these specific rituals biologically may be the only path to health in this way. Eating hudut is not only nourishing the body through the fresh herbs and nutrients it delivers: the practice of eating it also solidifies a person's Garifuna identity, allowing the space and time to embody "Garifuna-ness." Like the Kriol Belizeans in Texas, members of this community seek ways to "replenish their Belizeaness" and create transnational "assemblages" of what it means to be Belizean and, in this case, to be Garifuna.[10] Eating hudut means replenishing identity through cultural practice described in biological terms. The accuracy of the genetic explanation for food preferences and practices aside, the cultural and the biological intersect in the sensory experience of preparing hudut. The soreness in the arms from working the giant, wooden mortar and pestle to mash the plantains; the sound of the cracking of the coconuts and the rub of their flesh along the small, hard pieces of shell embedded in the wooden grater; and the smell of the frying fish and herbaceous coconut broth boiling on the stove wafting through the house—these alter the body in ways that scientists are still beginning to understand but that Indigenous communities have long known and articulated.[11] Doing things a

---

10. Johnson (2019) discusses ways in which cultural identity is created through practice among Belizeans who lead transnational lives, moving between Belize and the United States.

11. "these alter the body in ways that scientists": In recent decades, the science around epigenetics, or how the genome, once understood to be fixed at conception, can change through events and practices that occur during the course of a life, has exponentially expanded. For detailed discussions on how developments in understanding epigenetic processes impact anthropological research, see Thayer and Non (2015), and—with a focus on the body—Lock (2015), and—with a focus on structural inequalities and biases—Dressler et al. (2012), and—adding a neuroanthropological focus—Lende (2012), and—with a focus on biological mechanisms—Tung and Gilad (2013). See Noble (2013) for a discussion from a physiological perspective, explicitly engaging with the fixed, genetic explanations for behavior prominent in biological discourse. "that Indigenous communities": The EEH framework (Baines 2016a, 2018) seeks to capture the ways that Indigenous communities know that bodies

certain way, feeling them a certain way, changes the body—and is critical to health.

TOGETHER WE ARE MORE

"She really needed her earrings. They were really important to her, and once I found them, she felt so much better. She started doing so much better." The nursing home attendant had noticed my earrings and was explaining to me about an elderly Maya woman who came to the home without any of her traditional clothes, including her earrings. At the urging of several community members in Santa Cruz, I had bought myself earrings in the "traditional Maya" style, recognizable throughout Belize, almost a decade earlier, and was still wearing them. I had come to the nursing home to visit Marciana, who, at ninety-seven, had needed to finally move from the green-and-white house in Dangriga. She now lived here in San Ignacio, one of the larger Belizean towns on the western border. The nursing home, like the town, was home to older people of mixed ethnicity, with Marciana being in the Garifuna minority and sharing the airy, tropical space with Maya, Q'eqchi', Kriol, Mestizo, and other elders. The first time I visited, Marciana was participating in a Catholic prayer service with her friends. Representatives from all Belizean ethnicities traditionally practice Catholicism, most notably among Maya and Garifuna communities. Researching traditional practices has frequently taken me into Catholic homes, as these are often considered to be those that have retained most of their heritage practice, perhaps ironically through the church, which is often the venue for traditional music and dance across Garifuna and Maya communities.

---

change through practice in the lifecourse. For more on how Indigenous ways of knowing are reflected in epigenetic discourse, see Ko'omoa and Maunakea (2017), and—with a discussion of the political implications of the recognition of this intersection—Warin, Kowal, and Meloni (2020). For a comprehensive discussion of the overlap between indigenous ways of knowing and medical science, see Redvers (2019).

Back in Brooklyn, the songs performed in church are central to Garifuna language preservation, just as in Santa Cruz the playing of the marimba, a traditional wooden instrument, in church is fundamental to its continued relevance. The conversation about the traditional earrings, followed by this reminder of the place of the church in relation to traditional practice, served as a welcome reminder of how these practices were valued in Belize, even in the somewhat clinical setting of a nursing home.

After the short, outdoor service, Marciana and I visited until she was called in to dinner. Helping to serve the meal, I noticed that the residents had slightly different plates of food. The Maya woman, who now had her earrings so fundamental to her identity, was served corn tortillas, which I have learned over many years are "what Maya people eat."[12] Marciana had cassava in her soup—a tuber eaten across Belize (and many of the world's communities living on that latitude) but especially important in Garifuna cooking. Other residents were offered a choice between bread and flour tortillas. Chicken provided the thread across all the meals. When I remarked on how impressed and appreciative I was that the home provides such culinary diversity, the nurse explained that well-fed people equal happy people. She went on to share with me the experiences and observations that have led her to conclude that health is most closely linked with emotional well-being. While foods nourish the body, they are also very closely linked to heritage and identity, and connecting with these is critical to being well. Eating and worshiping in community is important for the elderly residents to stay healthy, but connecting with their culinary heritage is a critical piece of their wellness maintenance.

"We experience good health because we come together to talk." Back in Brooklyn, I was sitting at a table with Rosita and several other Garifuna ladies representing not only Belize but also the other recognized countries of the Garifuna diaspora:

---

12. See Baines (2016a), chap. 3, "Nutrition as Tradition: 'It's What Indian People Eat,'" for a full discussion of the links between food and Maya identity in southern Belize.

Honduras, Guatemala, and Nicaragua. They were ready and waiting to lead the opening procession at an event celebrating St. Vincent, the ancestral homeland of Garifuna people. We were discussing the role of Garifuna traditions in maintaining health. Rosita continued, "It would be difficult, as I see it, for you to do the traditions without the language. When we go to a traditional Garifuna activity, our songs are in Garifuna, our prayers are in Garifuna, the names of our food are in Garifuna." The Garifuna language was playing an important role in this event through the songs of the procession and the dances, its use being a traditional practice.[13] As the ladies prepared to begin their procession, I went to check out the room. Around the perimeter of the event space, vendors had set up small tables to sell traditional products. I was drawn to a table with attractive woven baskets presided over by hip Garifuna young people. I noticed that the baskets were filled with traditional herbs: lemongrass and others similar to those Rosita finds at the Korean shop under the subway. Their beautiful packaging, with names in both English and Garifuna, seemed to fit perfectly into the reimagining of the Brooklyn aesthetic. The historically Caribbean neighborhoods in Brooklyn were in the midst of ongoing gentrification, with what might have once been considered as outdated or underdeveloped now being repackaged to appeal to a young professional "hip" demographic. In this space where the mundane and the celebratory converged, the fluid nature of heritage became clear, as did the many ways, both subtle and obvious, that heritage manifests in the body. As one of the ladies clearly summarized in a later conversation, "take care of your mind, body, and soul; try to be stress-free, drink herbs, do your traditions."

In March 2020, coming together to talk, to cook, to sing took on a different meaning. During the COVID-19 pause order in New York City, which prohibited social gatherings, I spoke to Rosita

---

13. I would learn later when I traveled there that very few people in St. Vincent speak Garifuna. Details of the Garifuna homecoming trip to Yurumein (St. Vincent and the Grenadines) can be found in chapter 5 and in a forthcoming article.

on the phone. She was safe in her home and expressed frustration at what she saw as an individualistic mindset reflected in the behavior of others: "We don't need no Supreme Court to tell us what to do. We're human beings for God's sake!" Over the years that followed, I witnessed that different Garifuna people expressed a focus on the value of collectivity, particularly on my social media feeds. For example, a 2020 Facebook post featuring Garifuna anthropologist and author E. Roy Cayetano shared that it is the collective as opposed to the individual good that matters, articulating the Garifuna phrase *au bun amürü nu*: "I for you and you for me." This concept resonates with Indigenous and Afro-descended worldviews across time and space and echoes in the Mopan Maya saying *usk'inak'in*, which translates to "a day for a day" and refers to the reciprocal practice of helping each other plant and harvest corn, and *komonil* in Q'eqchi' Maya, which means the practice of coming together to share in collective decision-making and practice. In Belizean Kriol communities one similarly hears *wan wan okro ful baaskit*, which translates to "one one okra full basket" and refers to each person making a small contribution, creating enough for everyone. While I had always documented and felt the ways in which different groups had articulated how ecological practices were connected to health and wellness, in the social media space the links between these communities became increasingly clear. I thought back to something Rosita had said that very first time we sat down together. Talking about the Maya and Garifuna communities in Belize, she reminded me that "they live as one. It would be difficult for the government to pull them apart. They've been living together for many, many years. They didn't just start that yesterday."

"THEY DON'T KNOW WHAT THEY'VE GOT"

I was sitting in the offices of the Toledo Alcaldes Association in Punta Gorda in 2022 when I heard the news that Marciana had peacefully passed away. She was one hundred. A few days later, I made my way to Dangriga to meet Rosita in her mother's green house by the water tank. She was waiting for my arrival, looking down from that second-story balcony in the same way as her mother had those years before. We were old friends in New York City, but this was the first time she and I had shared time and space in Belize. We sat on the balcony with the sea just out of view, but the sea breeze on our skin, grateful in the Caribbean summer. Family and friends came by to sit awhile, pay respects, and share stories of Marciana's long and rich life. My favorite was how she walked to her farm two miles away every day well into her nineties. She had planted cassava, okra, plantains, and so much more, and would tend to her plants carrying her harvests home. They had convinced her, relatively recently, to take a taxi on the way home, because the roots she had dug were heavy. Her grandson who shared this story with me talked about using this family land for a farming venture, maybe growing peppers for the local hot sauce company. Like the taxi driver I had spoken to in the same green house several years before, he spoke about some of the younger generation hoping to relearn and reimagine the relationship their families traditionally had with local plants. "Change has to come from within," he said, referring to the distance many young Garifuna have from their heritage practices. He moved back to Dangriga after a successful career in the United States, his decision heavy with the internal dialogue about what it means to live a good life. I relished in the stories about Marciana's long, good life, having already known something of how she embodied her relationship with plants, the land, and her Garifuna heritage, but I was fascinated by how her relatives articulated their relationships to these same practices through the lens of returning to Dangriga to celebrate and remember her life.

 Rosita asked me to join her on a walk around town to pick up a few supplies for the house and the upcoming funeral service. On our way to the market for some fresh fruits, we passed under an almond tree, our flip-flopped feet stepping in and around the mashed fruits that had dropped and been left on the path to rot. She shook her head a little as she contemplated the wasted food. "You have to leave it to see it; the people who live here, they don't even know what they got." As we passed the small fenced yards, she pointed out the different plants poking through onto the sidewalk—there was the one to treat the sores, and over there, the cerasee to clean the blood.

When we reached the shore, she introduced me to her brother-in-law, who sat in the sea breeze amid the wood shavings making a drum for his daughter, who had recently started to learn to play traditional Garifuna drums. I asked them if there had been any pushback about women playing, drums having traditionally been played by men, and they said no. This pleased me, and I thought about change in the context of the fluidity of Garifuna heritage. The embodied practice of making the drum—the smoothing of the curves of the base, the smell of the freshly carved wood mixing with that of the salty ocean, the rustling palm trees punctuated by the dramatic swoops and dives of the fishing frigate birds—all this has changed very little. However, the practice is learned and reimagined by the next generation of Garifuna musicians.

Music is central to the articulation of Garifuna heritage, and music and dance appear at most every gathering, whether a small church service or larger celebration. While not unusual across cultures, both in Belize and beyond, Garifuna music has served as central to the identity of the Garifuna in Belize and has its own role in the cultural representation of the nation of Belize.[14] Large Garifuna drums mark the entrance to Dangriga, reminding visitors of this legacy—and its role in the present day. Garifuna music and dance, explored further in chapter 5, serves as both a place of storytelling, with new lyrics being written across the diaspora to share traditional stories with children in

---

14. In 2001 Garifuna music, language, and dance were proclaimed a "Masterpiece of the Oral and Intangible Heritage of Humanity" by UNESCO. The revival, maintenance, and international visibility of Garifuna music in Belize is, in large part, credited to songwriter Andy Palacio and his band, the Garifuna Collective.

this form, and also a site of the embodiment of both the fluidity and the consistency of heritage practice.

LIFE GOES ON

The palm trees rustled in the wind again as we sipped our drinks, overlooking the white sand free of seaweed and raked smooth. We had come to dinner at one of the oldest resorts in Dangriga. Rosita and her family had been here many times over the years, but I, never having been, was the one who had suggested it. Marciana had sold her cassava pudding to the resort, I learned, and they could not get enough to keep up with demand, because it had a reputation for being that good. Even though it also attracted foreign visitors, Belizeans came here too, and the owners were local people, which seemed reassuring after the negative effects of the increase in foreign investment in beach resorts further along the coast in Hopkins and Placencia. I was generally curious about the place, but I wanted to come primarily to meet up with a young woman from Santa Cruz who I had heard worked there. I had known her when she was growing up and was close with her family. Young people from the village working in Dangriga was a recent change. I wanted to see how she was doing with the change, particularly in the wake of the tragic and unexpected loss of her older brother. He had been just months away from being the first university graduate from Santa Cruz when he passed away. I knew him as an excellent student and a kind and thoughtful young man, and had spent some time talking about him with their parents just the previous week, I told her. His mother had relayed that on his last trip back to Santa Cruz from the university he had gone to the farm with her and helped her to pick beans. He never forgot he was Maya, his family, his traditions, she said. Sitting at the table with us, his sister shared how she had decided to work for a while and save some money before she went to university. She always admired her brother and wanted to follow directly in his footsteps, but now, in her grief and confusion, that path was less clear. As she left the table and went about her night, we finished our meals, and my companions remarked about how intelligent, thoughtful, and beautiful they found her to be. I nodded, the breeze and the conversation calling me back to my body and the present, not away from the two particular people we had just lost in the very recent past but toward a collective understanding of how the past does not need to be lost in the construction of the future. We carry it with us, in our bodies, in our practices, into a well future together.

CHAPTER 4

"YOUR MONEY WILL KILL YOU, ONE TIME"

A FEW MONTHS LATER IN 2022, I was back in Santa Cruz visiting with Jose Mes, a longtime friend and collaborator who had held several leadership positions in the village over the past decade. As I entered his familiar house on the hill at the entrance of the village, he greeted me in a jovial Mopan "*Biki lech*? (How are you?)" and then quickly followed up with "Have you had your caldo yet?" The immediacy of this question was not altogether unusual and reflected the importance of eating the traditional soup in reconnecting with the goings-on in the village, as if it in some way restored my "Mayaness" or my critical understandings of being Maya and my connections to the community. Most importantly, eating caldo ensures that I am, and will remain, well. I felt his question implied I had been out of the village for a few months and needed a healthy recharge. I assured him that my good friends on the other end of the village were building a new house that morning and that I had already had caldo with them. I had helped to prepare it to feed those who were lashing together the tall sticks to create the frame of the home. I had been charged with peeling the many small cloves of local garlic and washing and chopping the herbs: *samat* (culantro), harvested from the grassy areas around the house and cilantro, bought at the market.[1] I handed my prepped items to older women in the room, who added them to the huge boiling pot on the hearth, already red with the *k'uxub* (achiote) and glistening with the fat from local chickens, killed just hours before. It had been several months since I had a bowl of caldo and, as I stood and watched the soup boil, the garlic and herbs began to infuse with the aromas of woodsmoke and roasting corn masa of the tortillas made on the comal by the side of the pot, imparting a certain feeling of home. Some things don't change.

CHICKEN SOUP FOR THE MIND, BODY, SOUL

Standing over the pot that day, later reinforced by Jose's greeting, I thought about the significance of eating a bowl of caldo. One might say that it is symbolic, representing Maya hospitality, Maya traditions, Maya values. When someone visits a Maya home, or gives labor to a Maya family, they are given a bowl of caldo. It can be seen as a symbol of life, of gratitude. It is, in one sense, the most mundane or typical food but also the most special, often chosen for birthday celebrations and weddings. Essentially chicken soup (caldo can be made with ingredients other than chicken, notably pork, wild game meat, cassava or jippi jappa; however, chicken remains the most common and traditional ingredient), the importance of caldo in the maintenance of health is mirrored across many cultures and communities. Even in the most biomedically oriented communities, Grandma's chicken soup is prescribed for colds and other illnesses.[2] Watching the pot boil and the bubbling soup consume the bright

---

1. Culantro, or *Eryngium foetidum*, is an herb and medicinal plant similar and taste to cilantro but visually very different, with wide, flat, long leaves.

2. The biological analysis of the composition of chicken soup has shown its health benefits, particularly therapeutic in combating invading microbes associated with illness. For an analysis of chicken soup, and

green herbs, pulling them into its depths, I recognized that the soup was certainly rich with healthy nutrients for the body while also being a symbol of Maya identity; however, there was more to its connection to wellness, a deeper connection that brought together the biological and the social through the embodied practice of chopping herbs and cleaning chickens and tending the fire and stirring the massive pot. Preparing, sharing, and eating caldo was where the social became biological.

I thought back to my experience with the making of hudut in Brooklyn. When Jose asked me if I had had my caldo, he did not say, "It's in our DNA," but the language of caldo is quite similar. Declarations such as "It's what Maya people eat" evoke an understanding that, like Garifuna connections to hudut, Maya connections to caldo are somehow fundamental to the essence of identity. Watching women make the soup, the careful unspoken movements, the timing of the added ingredients, nothing measured, only felt, the careful dishing up and serving, it is easy for visitors to use the language of genetics, "It's in their DNA!" It is clear that there is an assumption among community members that the sensory experience of making and eating caldo in this sense is embodied not just by those who are Maya but also by people like me who have spent a long time in Maya communities. There is an assumption that the practice of making and eating caldo changes people's bodies, and once they have experienced that change, they will now always need caldo to remain well. In this sense, there is an assumption that a body—perhaps even one's DNA—has changed through the embodied practice. I thought back to what Anthony and Isaiah had told me about needing their caldo when they returned to Santa Cruz. Many of the young people who have worked out of the village in Caye Caulker and other tourist centers, including Jose's eldest son, have referred to coming home to eat caldo as well. True, young people often make a point of enjoying rice and flour tortillas and barbeque—more pan-Belizean foods. However, while the

---

other "folk remedies" from the perspective of teaching microbiology, see Fuller and Torres (2021).

narratives around caldo being essential to health might change, many still make a point to eat it when they come home.

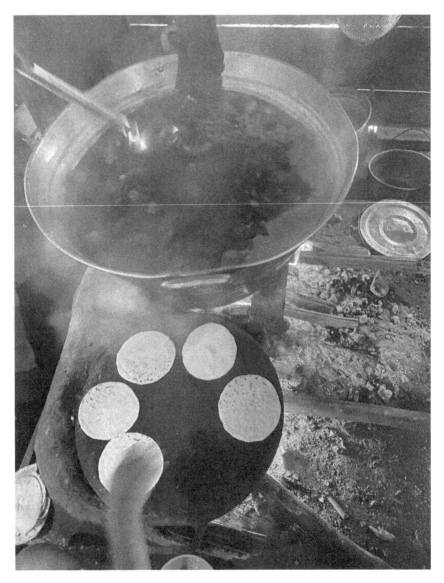

FIGURE 7 Preparing caldo and tortillas on the fire hearth. Santa Cruz village, Toledo, Belize. Kristina Baines.

PRACTICING CLIMATE CHANGE: SCIENTIFIC RHETORIC AND FARMING SUCCESS

Having reassured him about my fortification with caldo that morning, I went on to talk with Jose about how his oldest son, Wilmer, was still working out of the village but had decided to come back to Santa Cruz to get married. He already had his own farm. Jose had always encouraged his children to study and work outside of the village; however, he also made sure that he taught all of them how to farm, making the point to me many times over the years that he felt it was critical for them to have this knowledge to come back to. Wilmer had been working to save money to attend university. In previous years, Jose had told me that Wilmer wanted to study science, but a science degree was too expensive, so he had switched to a less-expensive degree path that "was still science." Assuring me that the degree was "still science" seemed to be aimed to appeal to my Western academic sensibilities. Perhaps he assumed or internalized through his many years of working with Western academics and business owners that I held science in higher regard than other subjects. He was adept at speaking what might be termed the "technical language of the colonizers," and, while I understood his knowledge to be vast across all domains, I knew him to be deeply rooted in what he would call "traditional" ecological practices. While he explained the significance of his son's new course of study, he made a point of relaying how Wilmer had just been home helping to clean the cacao field and plant the *matambre* (the dry season corn). I appreciated how explicit he was in valuing tradition in the context of robust engagement with the ideology and practices of external development processes, and I was always curious to learn about the embodied heritage practice through the lens of what he learned in his leadership capacity, attending trainings in and outside of the country on a wide range of topics, including farming practices, most recently in the context of climate change.

"Every plant I saw had come out." Jose was chatting to me in 2019 about his decision to change his farming practice from slash-and-burn to slash-and-mulch. He was the first person in Santa Cruz to try this new mulching technique. "I was talking to some friends, and it gave me an idea—two ways of farming," he said of his decision to make the change to the traditional agricultural practice. Slash-and-burn, known as swidden agriculture or shifting cultivation, had been the norm in subsistence farming communities in southern Belize for hundreds of years. In recent years, it had become one of the most controversial traditional practices for a variety of social and technical reasons. In this conversation, Jose told me how he was motivated to make the change because of drought. It was the first week in June, and the rains had only just started. Maya farming systems do not include irrigation systems, with farmers relying completely on the rains. Fields are typically chopped, burned, and planted in May, when they expect the rains to start. Many farmers had been talking about problematic changes in rainfall in recent years, many discussing how they might be related to climate change. When the weather is too dry, the mulched plant material retains moisture and makes sure the young plants do not dry out and perish, Jose explained. Also, there had been a lot of recent damage from fires burning out of control, with four acres of matambre corn and four acres of cacao accidentally burned the previous year. These fires create threatening situations, both environmental and social, and they signal more than just climate change. Elders discussed how some youth and newcomers have not properly learned the traditional ways of controlling fires when preparing their fields for planting. Fires, when carefully set and maintained, are critical to healthy soil and healthy corn, I was told, supporting my "scientific" understanding about nitrogen release and soil fertility. And they were very much historically a part of Maya—and other—land management practices. Jose told me he respected the decisions of most of the farmers to burn because they know how to handle the fires; however, he has had great results from his switch to slash-and-mulch and has been sharing his experiences with his community. As rainfall continues to be unpredictable and conversations around climate change become more frequent, some community members are following suit. Others have weathered changes before, they say, and keep their practice of slash-and-burn, albeit with different modifications.

"Technology can open your mind; some people use it for anything bad." Later that year, I was on the other side of the village talking to some village elders about the changes they see in farming practices, when Sussano, the oldest of four brothers and among the first residents of Santa Cruz, told me this. While the "a little bit good, a little bit bad" attitude toward changes—broadly conceived under the notion of "development" or progress—is very common, the changes in the weather, coupled with a perceived increase in agricultural improvement projects offered by both government and nongovernmental organizations to community members to address farming within this context, have increased skepticism about the role of science and technology in improving livelihoods and offering increased well-being. I was sitting in a familiar thatch house near the flooded football field and noticed a pile of dried corn. The usual straw-colored husks of some ears were interspersed with something new: a deep reddish-purple husk. I was surprised. Sussano had been saving seeds for over fifty years, and this corn did not appear to come from his seeds. He explained, "This is our first time planting *box holoch*, the seed we kept from before [with the straw-colored husk only]; the breeze came and blew it all away."[3] Hybrid corn seed is not uncommon in the village; however, it is more often used by younger farmers who either do not have saved seed or who are embracing the promise of the new hybrid technology.[4] While studies have found that technologically enhanced seeds do not necessarily guarantee higher productivity, the narrative

---

3. Translates to "dark husk."

4. Hybrid is defined here as created from the standard interbreeding of corn varietals to produce seeds sold locally. It should be noted that Maya farmers in southern Belize explicitly reject the use of GMO corn seeds. These were initially rejected throughout the entire country but have since been integrated into use by communities farming in some central areas of the country.

of better living through "science" is pervasive, especially among the younger generations.[5] While discussing the increased winds on that day, Sussano also shared additional insight into the reasons that some farmers were struggling with their corn yields. He noted that the younger farmers did not want to use candles or burn incense anymore, that there was nobody carrying on these practices, and that nobody was learning the traditions.[6] They were not doing the blessings and offerings to the hills, mountains, valleys. That's why there was no corn.

Sussano's assessment resonated with me as I later sat discussing the intersection of technology, tradition, and health with a young farmer who had planted hybrid seeds for about five years. He told me that he did not see anything wrong with burning incense while you planted corn seeds, that he understood that it was a tradition the old people liked to do and that it was not a bad or negative practice (even though his Baptist church would deem it as such), but he would not bother doing it because it does not actually *do* anything. It doesn't *actually* make the corn healthier. He chuckled, his smile tinged with a knowing glance shared with me, as he assumed I would agree that the agricultural science around corn crop success had nothing to do with burning incense. I was not as sure as he assumed I was. While I had not engaged in the systematic assessment of corn yields in relation to the ritual practices traditionally associated with planting, I had assessed the significance of burning incense to the overall wellness of individuals and families who engaged in the practice.[7] And it was significant. Burning incense was actually one the most significant practices linked to wellness. If it had the potential to increase wellness in the people involved in

---

5. For a discussion of the impacts of both corn seed varietals and soil fertility on corn yields see Cortez (2017) and Peller (2021).

6. Resin harvested from the copal tree is traditionally used as incense in ritual practices, like planting corn, and special ceremonies, almost exclusively among families who identify as Catholic.

7. See statistics in Baines (2016b), The Environmental Heritage and Wellness Assessment.

the planting, tending, and processing of the corn, it follows that it may possibly increase the health of the corn itself. I did not tease out the particular mechanisms of the embodied practice, the sensory pathway through which the smell of incense is processed through the hippocampus and evokes memories, which are processed in the same part of the brain. The enskilling of farmers, and the embodied knowledge they carried with them, could clearly be linked to the activation of those memories in the brain through this process.[8] Thus, the ritual associated with the planting, which included the burning of incense, was critical to activating the farmers in such a way that they would be more likely to plant a successful field of corn.

"I am not a climate scientist, but I can comfortably say to you that the Maya farmers of southern Belize are not responsible for the global climate crisis." It was two pandemic years later, in 2022, and I was in a neighboring village facilitating a workshop on the most important Maya traditions to practice for healthy people, healthy communities, and healthy forests.[9] A participant shared that they heard from the facilitators of a previous workshop that the burning associated with the practice of slash-and-burn has a negative impact in terms of generating the increased temperatures associated with climate change, and that Maya farmers are causing the problem. Frustrated, I offered my definitive response and described how corporate carbon emissions far exceed anything generated by traditional Maya farming practices. My frustration was not with the farmers, who were sincere in their efforts to incorporate new strategies to maintain livelihoods in a changing world, but with the organizations who offer technical support and training around faulty assumptions

---

8. Ingold (2021) makes a detailed argument for "enskillment": "Neither innate nor acquired, skills are grown, incorporated into the human organism through practice and training in an environment. They are thus as much biological as cultural."

9. This workshop was part of a project of the Toledo Alcaldes Association facilitated by the Julian Cho Society. See Baines and Miis (2024) for more details.

and logics. In this case, the logics were easily challenged, even by their own frame of reference. Back over the farmer's road at Jose's house, he was telling me about his latest response to climate challenges. He said he still used slash-and-mulch in his cornfields, instead of slash-and-burn, but he explained how he had been learning about permaculture principles. His use of the language of permaculture was curious, and even he noted that growing crops and raising local animals together in the ways permaculture encourages is exactly what Maya people have always done. Jose and I have had many conversations over the years about how some people in "developed" countries such as the United States have been returning to more small-scale and sustainable farming methods as the multiple dimensions of the destructive nature of the industrial food system have revealed themselves.[10] The interface with the Western scientific language and concepts that Jose just employed may actually not obscure the value of traditional practice but rather make traditional Maya agriculture legible in a wider frame of environmental activism, moving beyond southern Belize into spaces of government and NGO work where it might have previously been dismissed as irrelevant or archaic. While it may be easy to bemoan the necessity of this legibility, it is an important step in recognizing what it means for heritage to be processual. Traditional practices are a lived experience rather than a somehow precious, static entity waiting to be preserved. Recognizing this is a critical step in understanding how change is negotiated.

WORKING TOGETHER: THE MOST IMPORTANT MAYA TRADITION TO KEEP

"They don't know how to thatch anymore. They are going to school, and they don't want to give the free labor anymore." Sussano's complaints about the younger generation take a similar

---

10. For a detailed critique of the industrial food system and the changes to diets it has precipitated, see Wood et al. (2023).

tone to that of grandparents around the world, a bemoaning of the changes they see in the youth, a nostalgic callback to all that was better before those changes. In this case, all my time spent in southern Belize has taught me that the loss of the reciprocal labor system is actually, quite rightly, cause for concern. It is not just the elders who discuss the value of reciprocity. Working together to plant and harvest corn, cook meals for celebrations, and build houses is a traditional practice that provides central social and economic benefits critical to a healthy Maya life. While the reciprocal labor system—in which community members provide a day of work for their neighbors on request and those neighbors then owe them a day of labor in the future—is what people generally mean when they use the English phrase "working together," this practice has come to symbolize not just the embodied practice but a wider acknowledgment of wider Maya values related to collective decision-making and rotating community leadership. As the village governance processes interface with those of the nation-state, Maya leaders have made a concerted effort to strengthen the collectivist approach through bolstering the decision-making capacity of alcaldes, who in turn listen to both community members in formalized village meetings and other alcaldes as part of the Toledo Alcaldes Association. Villages continue to hold fahinas, albeit with varying degrees of frequency and participation, when community members come together to work to clean and maintain the common areas in the village, around the community center and the school, for example. Participation in the fahina is an obligation of village membership; however, alcaldes note an increase in the numbers of people who send the small amount of money required in case of absence.

The replacement of cash for reciprocity and community labor is problematic in the economic sense, because cash flow is rarely steady; however, the concerns run deeper than this. When the health of an individual body is understood in terms of how it moves through an ecological system, and this movement—or the practices that form this movement—are explicitly collectivist, threats to the system are threats to the individual body. These threats can be clearly material in nature; for example, if not enough people are willing to help plant corn, a farmer can either plant less corn, thus providing less food for his self and his family, or he can do more work by himself, becoming overworked and fatigued. If there are no young people willing to help with processing corn, the farmer may need to eat more food from the shop, which is less nutritious. Additionally, the erosion of working together as a value erodes the possibilities for engaging with the landscape in ways deemed traditional; it disconnects community members from the practices of being in the world as a Maya person. Changes happen in communities and ecological systems, but without collective approaches, how are individuals able to stay well amid the changes?[11] As the community leader and activist Pablo Miis summarized community reports of identifying the practice of working together as a critically important tradition to keep, "This has to come first; without this, we cannot do anything else."

THE LANGUAGE OF MAYA VALUES: ETHNOBOTANICAL PRACTICE AND BIOSCIENCE

"*Cu wech walak o bet ti kech ti muk'a'anetch?*" My Mopan skills were rusty, but that sentence still rolled off my tongue with ease. "What makes a person healthy?" I had asked it so many times over the previous decade that I would never forget it. Nevertheless, the primarily Maya audience chuckled at my clumsiness, and I caught Jose's eye. He was smiling back at me. We had gathered that day in 2019 in Punta Gorda at the request of the Maya leaders for an *ab'ink*, or listening session, during which academics from Belize, the United States, and Canada

---

11. Indigenous scholars, and scholars working closely with Indigenous communities, have written much on the importance of relationality in these communities, incorporating a critique and rethinking of the research process as it relates to relational practice. See Tynan (2021), Galla and Holmes (2020), and Wilson (2008).

had been asked to share their research insights with the Maya communities to serve their goals of articulating Maya priorities and values as part of healthy Maya livelihoods, in the context of the land rights articulation and implementation process. The academics for the most part felt honored to have been invited, excited that their research might be useful to the leaders and communities as they moved to promote and protect the values their community members deemed important. It seemed like this could be a step toward a kind of decolonial endeavor, working toward addressing the inherently extractive nature of academic research.[12] Many topics were discussed, including health, broadly defined and, more specifically in relation to the use of medicinal plants. Amid a lively discussion, participants stressed the need to protect the continuity of traditional medicinal practices but to take care not to freeze knowledge in time, understanding that it changes through dynamic practice. Respecting the protocols for learning the "bush doctor business" were stressed, with the proper training of interested young people forefronted.

Maya community members shared concerns that Indigenous peoples around the world had been experiencing a rush of interest in their traditional plant medicines—called "bush medicine" in Belize—by pharmaceutical companies who showed little respect for their intellectual property rights. The companies focused on isolation of the pharmacological properties of the plants while stripping them of the ritual context in which they are administered. A few years earlier, when the Maya healers of southern Belize had been in discussion about setting up a clinic in the coastal town next door to the hospital, they had asked some of the researchers working with them to isolate the pharmacological properties of the *chi'k'a* (gumbo limbo) in order to provide proof of the efficacy of their medicinal practice. The researchers did indeed find therapeutic efficacy in the isolated plant compounds in the lab, but Indigenous healers and others

---

12. For more analysis of the experiences of the *ab'ink*, and a detailed discussion of the process as a decolonial methodology, please see Baines (forthcoming), "Decolonial Methodologies: Lessons from the Ab'ink."

understood that chemical compounds are only part of the therapeutic story related to ethnobotanicals.[13] The ritual setting, the burning of incense, the singing, chanting, all are part of the sensory experience of healing. Even the most skilled traditional healers, however, are overtly conscious of the perceived need to eliminate all factors with the exception of the pharmacological components when discussing efficacy.[14] Like in the practice of planting corn, the ritual elements of the administration of the healing plant medicines is not simply a symbolic component but an embodied one.[15] The hope among the Maya healers was to "stay relevant" in the context of biomedicine, in part through isolating the chemical component of the medicines. I considered that it might behoove biomedicine to take seriously the relevance of the sensory components of therapeutic encounters. The "noise" or the "placebo effect" eliminated in drug trials is actually the meaning of these encounters.[16] When healing is "in the mind," it is also in the body.

As the conversation moved on, leaders considered the benefits of certification for the healers, of which the biopharmaceutical efficacy was only a part. The arguments for certification

---

13. This research is detailed in Walshe-Roussel (2014).

14. The RCT has gone some distance to instilling this pharmacological focus in the popular consciousness. Randomized Controlled Trials (RCTs) were first discussed in a 1948 paper, becoming the "gold standard" for testing pharmaceuticals in the 1980s. They involve isolating the pharmacological components of a particular drug by eliminating the placebo effect through administering either the drug or a placebo in a setting in which neither the researcher or the patient knows who receives the active compound. This is referred to as "double-blinding."

15. Hatala and Waldram (2015, 2017) detail how sensory experience and "emplotment" directly involve the roles of performance and social action in healing practice in southern Belize.

16. Moerman (2002) describes how the meaning in the healing process shifts in different populations and what we might describe as "placebo effects" are critical to those meanings and the efficacy of the healing process.

suggested that this would give them legitimacy in the spaces occupied by biomedical clinics and ensure they had followed a training process. The concern was that, like so many Indigenous practices, traditional healing modalities are fluid, and that there were not necessarily one or two data points to capture for certification. Community members cautioned against holding healers accountable to an incomplete or irrelevant standard. There was not one prevailing conclusion that day; however, the urgency behind continuing the conversation was noted.

"The doctors don't do anything; bush medicine is better." I was back in Santa Cruz later that year and a neighbor was crushing leaves to prepare a poultice to wrap on a friend's swollen ankle. As he carefully placed the leaves on the ankle, he continued his critique of biomedicine. It was one I was hearing more and more, particularly since the health clinic in the neighboring village opened about a decade ago, increasing engagement in the biomedical system by eliminating the barrier of travel to Punta Gorda. Critiques were many, and included miscommunication, injections, pills that did not address the issues, and lack of follow-up. Complaints about biomedicine, and this new health clinic that dispensed it, were many. The previous summer, another father had told me how his daughter had a fever and traveled to see a bush doctor after a week of no response from biomedicine. A young mother told me how she was going across to Guatemala to get an injection and would follow up with bush medicine if that was unsuccessful. Others were concerned about language barriers, cesarean sections performed with unclear rationales, and long waits for treatment. There were concerns about expense. Both the clinics and hospitals, and now some traditional healers, were charging more money than people had to spend, leaving confusion about how to prioritize health interventions. When I spoke about reasons for forest conservation with an older woman in a neighboring village, she stressed the monetary drivers, noting, "We need the forest because the plants we need for medicines are in there, and it's getting too expensive to go to the clinic."

The varied experiences of community members with medical care demonstrate that there is not a clear, catch-all solution for addressing health problems. However, it is clear that equitable access to biomedical clinics and their interventions is important to communities. In addition, and more important to many people, access to traditional ethnobotanical knowledge and trained healers is also a critical part of healthcare that should be maintained. Understanding the intersection of land management and traditional healing practice emerged from these conversations as vital in understanding this facet of how healthy bodies are connected to healthy forests. But the plants are just part of the story.

HERITAGE ON DISPLAY

"They need to go out and get a job; they are 24/7 on Facebook." It is 2019 in Santa Cruz, and a young Maya man shared a standard criticism of his peers and of the insidious nature of social media. While I did not disagree, I admitted that I enjoyed seeing more and more of the children I got to know a decade ago appearing on my social media platforms. I found joy in wishing them happy birthdays, celebrating as they got married and had children of their own. Amid the selfies and the twinkle heart emojis, I had also noticed a—perhaps unexpected—trend in celebrating traditional practices. Pictures of cacao fields and glistening bowls of caldo came across my feed. And these images did not just serve to keep me connected; they were helping Belizeans stay connected to their communities too. While use of social media was prevalent before the 2020–2021 pandemic hiatus, these images increased during that time. They also seemed to challenge the narratives of the loss of traditional practice among the youth in their own communities. As I was walking with a young university graduate in 2022 through her Maya village, she shared that she had never seen anyone play the "corn game" in her lifetime.[17]

---

17. The corn game is a game with similar principles to parcheesi played on the night before the May corn planting. During the game, incense and candles are burned near the bag of corn seed, serving as a blessing for the

I shared that I had only seen it once in all of my time in Belize. She had thought that nobody did it anymore until she saw her cousin post pictures on his feed of him and his friends playing it. Relaying the story, she was excited, hoping she would get to see it in person someday soon. Social media had made this practice visible and seemed to also add value or cachet in some way to a game that has otherwise been dismissed as "old-fashioned."

Several years previously, I had noticed more and more young people standing on the hill at the entrance to the village, catching cell service to watch, I later found out, YouTube videos. Around that same time, Basilio Teul, a longtime village leader, advocate for Maya values and longtime friend, asked me to support him in writing a grant to put on a Deer Dance in Santa Cruz. His goal was to include everyone in the community in celebrating in this traditional way. They would need funds to rent the costumes, and they would need substantial funds to offer meals to the entire village who he hoped would come to watch over the four days of the dance. As we collaborated on the budget, we considered ways in which young people could be engaged in learning about their traditions and decided to include funding for a documentary film to capture the Deer Dance and interviews with some of the dancers and other community members. As part of the filming, we included training for local students to learn to use the cameras and take part in the editing process. Our goals were multiple: Basilio was especially interested in documenting the dance for the dancers to watch themselves, with a mind to improving their skills and showing it to young dancers coming up. I imagined the young people standing on the hill and watching the Deer Dance between their streams of Beyonce and Jay Z. We received the funding, and, while the process was not without challenges, the dance took place, in

---

seed. A rich meal of pig intestine, lung and liver with hot corn tortillas is often served late in the evening after the game, fortifying the players and the cooks, who will both be working hard the next morning to plant and cook again for the after-planting meal.

January 2016.[18] We enjoyed four days of celebrations in Santa Cruz, and the film was made, capturing in time a snapshot of this important traditional practice.

As I climbed the hill behind the community center two years later, I heard the familiar melodic jangle of the marimba. I knew that the only marimba in Santa Cruz was housed at the other end of the village, and I walked toward the sound. When I stepped into the house, announcing myself and accepting the welcome inside, my eyes began to adjust to the darkness indoors, but I did not see at first where the music was coming from. I chatted for a while with the ladies seated in the hammocks, enjoying the coolness during a hot afternoon, and then poked my head into the room where the music seemed to be coming from. Seated cross-legged on a freshly swept mud floor was a small child, perhaps three or four years old, holding a cellphone. I peered over his shoulder and saw that he was watching the Deer Dance documentary. Excited, I returned to my conversation and asked his mother and grandmother if this was something he liked to watch often. They assured me that, yes, he watched it all the time. They had not been expecting my visit, so I accepted that this was not something staged to please me, and I went on to ask what they thought about the film. "It is good for them to know the marimba music. This is our music, the traditional music for the Maya people. And the Deer Dance is good to know; it's our culture, our traditions. The children should know it." It was not until later when I looked at my photo of such a small child looking at a screen that I paused to consider what so many people had shared with me about changes brought to the village with technology. Indeed, this was a little bit good and a little bit bad.

That same year, I had a conversation with another one-time village leader who had chosen to move with his family out of Santa Cruz to a village up the Southern Highway closer to the capital, Belmopan. I had known him foremost as part of the

---

18. Thank you to the Positive Legacy Foundation for supporting the Deer Dance. The documentary film, "Maya Deer Dance, Belize" directed by Daniel Velazquez, can be watched on YouTube.

family of four generations who played the marimba. I had spent many an evening dancing into the night as the three essential players moved rhythmically up and down the hand-carved wooden keys with their mallets, laughing with Ixna Juana, the grandmother of the family, as we held our skirts and twirled around to the steady, echoing notes drifting into the cool, damp night air. The power of repetitive music and dance to transform the body has been well described in scholarship, with communities around the world from the Kalahari Desert to the cathedrals of England using music to open their bodies and minds to restore energy, to receive spirits, to connect with each other.[19] While I did enjoy making tortillas, dancing to the marimba provided some of my favorite moments of participant observation.

Santa Cruz residents had long expressed concern that the knowledge of traditional musicians and dancers might soon be lost. While there were four generations of marimba players, the knowledge was isolated to one family. During my last visit in 2022, the great-grandfather had lost his sight and was no longer able to play. The children were not coming around to learn. During my conversation that day with the former village leader, he offered a potential solution to the waning interest in traditional music in the village. At the time, the solution was jarring and unexpected; however, since then, I have heard similar arguments from others, including members of Garifuna communities. He explained that there were more opportunities to play marimba in the village closer to the capital, because tourists regularly visited there because it was easy to get there, and they were interested to hear the traditional music. He could play with other musicians, younger musicians, and more often, because there were more opportunities for payment. Reimagining or reinvigorating traditional practices for tourists is certainly a

---

19. For discussions about the role of sensory practice associated with music and dance and their relationship with health, see the work of Laderman and Roseman (2016), Noone (2020) and Downey (2002). For discussions specific to the communities in the Kalahari, see Katz (1982, 1984).

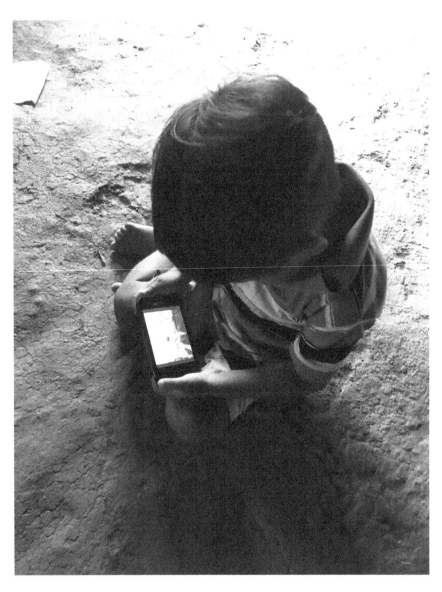

FIGURE 8 A young child watches the Deer Dance video. Santa Cruz village, Toledo, Belize. Kristina Baines.

widely discussed and contentious practice, bringing up questions of cultural commodification and power.[20] However, on that day, he painted a picture of Maya people from multiple communities coming together in their new village by the highway to play marimba into the night long after the tourist vans had gone back to their hotels. There was a river there too, he added, understanding its central role in the maintenance of Maya identity.

COME TO THE RIVER, GO TO THE FALLS

"This is her first time at the falls." Sonia, my longtime friend and younger sister to Jose, gestured at her young daughter who was happily making her way down the wide path at Rio Blanco National Park, a co-managed, sprawling swath of lowland forest with an impressive waterfall just a short walk from the village. I responded with surprise, but I wondered if that revelation had really surprised me. With the work of daily life taking up a lot of time and energy, visits to the waterfall are a luxury most often enjoyed by visitors, not villagers. I had spent much of my time in the village over the past decade doing daily work with Sonia, washing and bathing in the river being a significant part of that. While these particular forest paths had signs to mark the tree species and the falls in the river here were a little steeper, the park was simply an everyday ecosystem rather than a particular one, set aside to "go to" rather than simply "be in." Before the pandemic, in 2018, I had been asking questions about wellness practices in the area of the village around Sonia's house; as part of that research, I spoke to some younger women, who told me that going to visit the falls to "be in nature" made them happy. While this sentiment aligns with both anecdotal research and formalized scientific study, I, again, found it curious coming

---

20. For early discussions of cultural commodification and authenticity as they relate to Maya identity, see Medina (2003). For an overview of commodification as it relates to tourism from an anthropological perspectives, see Shepherd (2002).

from young people who grew up and lived their daily lives firmly "in nature."[21] This seemed like a narrative they had always known with their bodies, but the language they used seemed to have come from formal school settings. The "going to nature" narrative exemplified the separation of formalized learning in a school building from learning, and being in the environment has long been noted as a critique of the exporting of colonial curricula into schools across the world.[22]

As we bathed in the pools of the waterfalls, I thought about how many times Sonia and I had taken a swim in that same river. The paths to our washing spots were not as clearly marked as those at the national park, and she had worried for me, guiding my inexperienced feet across the slippery banks and mossy stones. "Mind you drop," she reminded me. It was important I did not fall, as doing so could be the source of a spectrum of grave injuries, even death, as had happened with a local mother just months before my arrival. Sonia too had suffered from a fall, which set off a chain of events that, she previously explained, had led to her difficulty in conceiving her first and only child. Sonia had ended up using medicinal plants found in the forests surrounding us to help in her healing and the conception of this child, who was now frolicking in pools with me. The biomedical system had offered little by way of explanation or help, so she had enlisted the assistance of a traditional healer. Some responses to interruptions in natural systems were found within the systems themselves. Sonia's healing journey made it clear to me in this moment that after a lifetime of taking bodies *to* nature, it seems an important reminder that our bodies *are* nature.

---

21. For a meta-analysis of cross-disciplinary research linking nature and happiness see Capaldi et al. (2014).

22. For a discussion of the way traditional learning practice happens in Maya communities in southern Belize, see Zarger (2010). For a discussion of the way nature is conceived as a place to "go to" in US school systems, see Baines (2001).

DO IT FOR MY VILLAGE, DO IT FOR LOVE

Hilda, another longtime friend and Jose's wife of twenty years, set down a steaming plate of sweet yams in front of me. It had been settled that I had already had my caldo, but Maya hospitality dictates that I should have something to eat while I talk. Ground food, yams, cassava, and other tubers grown underground in the forest and around the house are considered a healthy, local food, rich in nutrients and also traditional, an appropriate snack for me. As I eagerly dug into their soft, creamy flesh, Jose brought Hilda into our conversation. "She gives the turkeys bush medicine!" Hilda nodded, her impossibly wide smile broadening even further. The smile was tinged with a little embarrassment, even though my interest in and respect for traditional practice was widely known, especially in this household. I hoped this was changing, but I still regularly saw evidence of how years of being considered in some way "backward" or "less than" manifested in conversation with Indigenous communities, even in playful exchanges such as this one. It seemed that the years of formal and informal research on the efficacy of ethnobotanical medicines was still not enough to remove the stigma of the historical and ongoing delegitimization of Indigenous knowledge and practice. I responded enthusiastically as the turkeys wandered by, thinking about the antibiotics, hormones, and inhumane living conditions associated with US industrial poultry farming. The turkeys look great, I said, very healthy, very beautiful. *Kich'p'ana kutz.*

Resting in the hammock after my snack, I noticed a book on medicinal plants on a small shelf and pointed to it. Jose said of his son, Wilmer, then in his early twenties, "When he's here, when he's resting, he always loves to read that." I wondered for a minute if Jose was just trying to make me happy: Did this smart young person working out of his village really read about medicinal plants for fun when he was home visiting his family? Maybe this was part of his recharge along with eating caldo, I reasoned. Our conversation continued, and I asked about something Jose had said a few years back. The rains came early then, in February instead of May, and Jose had lost his crop of beans as a result. Around the same time, he was feeling frustrated with how much lobbying of politicians he was needing to do in his elected leadership role. He wanted to do right by his village and work to get them the resources they needed, but he felt the tensions of interfacing with wider Belizean politics. He had always said yes to opportunities, for himself, for his family, for his village and had a lot of experience dealing with the many facets of the pervasive cultural and economic systems associated with capital and hierarchy. Working hard, after all, is an important Maya value. Today, he seemed a little less tired and depleted, but he reinforced the sentiment that he shared with me those years ago: "Don't work because of money—do things for love, to have a happy life . . . your money will kill you, one time." It was then that he shared that Wilmer had decided not to go to university but to come back, get married, and work in service of his village. Although I knew Wilmer as a very promising young student, I nodded in understanding. Working for others is rarely an exercise in the pursuit of health and happiness.[23] The same week as Wilmer's wedding in May 2023, Santa Cruz hosted another Deer Dance, this time in collaboration with Belize Tourist Board's annual Cacao Fest celebration, a big change and a departure from the village-level dances in the past. The dancers shared their skills with visitors from around Belize and around the world, donning the pale-faced masks of the generals, mocking the colonial enterprise while celebrating the animals of the forest. Disentangling the traditional music and dance from its commodification in the context of Belizean tourist economies is difficult, and perhaps not even a useful enterprise. It is better perhaps to focus on the experience of the dancers and the spectators. In the music, in the moment, is the practice for money or for love? Or for health? Or for all of these?

---

23. For foundation discussions of wage work, see Marx's (1844) writings on alienation and the continued scholarly critique and discussion of his work.

CHAPTER 5

"SHE IS MY DOCTOR, SHE DANCE PUNTA"

I WAS STILL ON THE small, white tourist bus when I saw a flurry of activity out the window. Several of the ladies were moving quickly toward a hedge next to the snack stand in the waterfall parking lot. I heard delighted squeals as they reached the hedge area, heads nodding and hands moving about. When I disembarked and reached the hedge, peering into the circle, I quickly recognized what the fuss was about. "Cerasee!" Growing on the hedge was a vine, bitter melon, or cerasee, a wild plant common around tropical areas of the world. In Belize, it is used by many people, including those in both Garifuna and Maya communities, as a medicinal tonic, to clean the blood of toxins and purify the body. The ladies were removing the vine and wrapping it up in small bundles to carry with them and later boil to make the medicine. The delight at seeing the vine was amplified both by the fact that our contingent had traveled from New York City together, where most of us made our homes (the others having first traveled from Los Angeles), and where cerasee does not grow, and by the specific location and trip we were coming to the end of on that day. The group was traveling for a homecoming trip to St. Vincent, or Yurumein, the ancestral

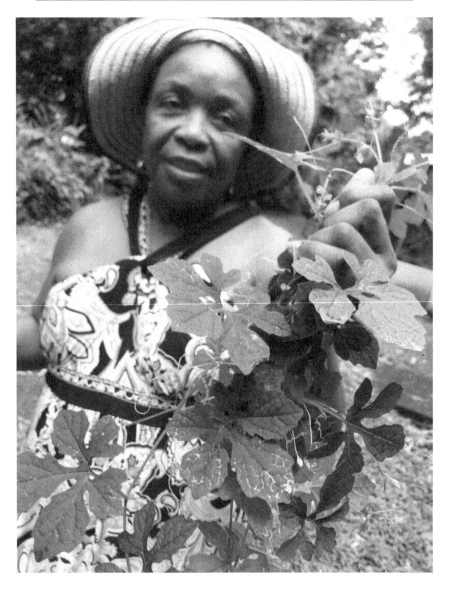

FIGURE 9 Rosita Alvarez with recently harvested cerasee vine (*Momordica charantia*). Yurumein (St. Vincent). Kristina Baines.

home of the Garifuna people. The 2019 contingent was made up of primarily Belizean Garifuna women living in either New York City or Los Angeles who, with a few exceptions, were visiting the island for the first time. The government of St. Vincent had collaborated with the organizers and Belizean governmental representatives from the United States to organize a variety of cultural activities around the island, most notably a trip via catamaran to Balliceaux, the small uninhabited island off the coast of the main island where the British exiled the Garifuna people in 1797, thus continuing their history of colonial genocide and dispossession and necessitating their subsequent resilience as they settled throughout the coastal Caribbean.

HERITAGE AS HOME

"Maybe that's why we kept our culture, because they left." Rosita somehow finds a grateful lens through which to engage with her history. Had the Garifuna not been forcibly removed from their homeland, and those who survived the years on Balliceaux not been sent to Roatan, and then scattered in settlements around the Caribbean, she may not have been compelled to keep up her cultural practices. Indeed, if she had not moved to Brooklyn from Belize, perhaps she would be engaged in her culture even less. She has expressed this sentiment to me many times, but here in Yurumein, in conversation with both her relatives and friends living in Los Angeles, and with the small community on the island who identify as Garifuna, it seems even more profound. Extreme change or disruption can crystallize deeply held values, practices that are protective across all dimensions of health, providing security, comfort, the necessary knowledge and skills to live, binding people to each other who can understand and help in times of need. Without the disruptive forces, perhaps it is easy to take for granted the everyday aspects of cultural practice, to lose sight of their value.

As our little tour bus struggled up the steep hills into the dense forests of the northern part of St. Vincent, I was reminded of the many struggles I had climbing the hills in the forests that are home to the Maya of southern Belize in the old white truck before the road was paved. Just as I would often have to do with my Maya friends in Belize, the driver here in St. Vincent asked those who could to get out and walk, promising we could rejoin at the top of the hill. "We are learning with our bodies!" I offered with a smile as a comment on our discomfort. By the time we reached the small Garifuna village that day, we had indeed gained some embodied knowledge about how and why this was the place where the small numbers of Garifuna remained. I felt at home in the small, Indigenous village in the tropical forest, my body being used to the uneven terrain and the dark, breezy coolness of the houses from my time spent in southern Belize. The group remarked on how the clay ovens in the houses used to bake bread with arrowroot were similar to those they were familiar with from baking cassava bread. The processing equipment also revealed a similar process to the traditional ways of processing cassava, with which my companions were very familiar. As we stepped from house to house, I wondered how my companions felt being simultaneously so close and so far away from these roots.

"We are able to bring the culture back to you!" Later in the week, we met some youth in a historically Garifuna, now mixed, village closer to the capital, where the contingent gave some lessons on Garifuna language songs and dance.[1] The language had been nearly lost, with the remaining Garifuna, like so many persecuted and marginalized Indigenous communities around the world, having hidden their identities through assimilation. It was only in recent years that a renewed interest in celebrating Garifuna culture and heritage traditions emerged here. Efforts at making Indigenous histories and present-day contributions visible are not unique to the Garifuna or to St. Vincent. Here, the phenomenon could be understood as a convergence of pan-Indigenous pride, political positioning, and economic opportunism, particularly in relation to tourist dollars from the United States. Pausing in front of the community center on that day, an older woman from Los Angeles got goose bumps as she talked

---

1. For a detailed discussion of the teaching of Garifuna culture through song and dance, see Myrtle Palacio's (2023) presentation from the Belize Kulcha symposium.

about how her parents had told her stories of this village, passed down as part of their histories. Standing in the place of those histories, she felt home, even though it had been hundreds of years since anyone in her family had been there.

We were swimming in the ocean off the coast of Balliceaux in a joyous escape from the island heat, an activity that I was happy to take part in even if I did not know if it was appropriate for a location so solemn and sacred. Another of our group who grew up and lived in Los Angeles shared with me that she was always reminded by her parents of her indigeneity. She explained how they hung pictures of American Indians in her home, and she saw them as ancestors. This is a different narrative from many Garifuna living in Los Angeles, who I have learned from many people more often lean into the West African part of their cultural heritage. Perhaps it is easier to be of mixed African and Indigenous ancestry in New York City, where communities of various Afro-Caribbean identities are plentiful and blended heritage is perceived as more normative.[2] It is easier for Californian kids to just say they are Black Americans, an identity that is more legible in the wider context of Los Angeles, and, of course, also true. Many older community members see this as a loss, many even as an affront to Garifuna culture and values as a whole, which they see as critical to a healthy, happy life. Bathing in the warm waters of the Caribbean Sea, my companion explained that, unlike some of her fellow pilgrims, she did not feel sad visiting Balliceaux. To her, this was a celebration of the strength and resilience of her ancestors rather than a mourning of their deaths. Historical trauma has been shown to be carried in different ways by different people in different places.[3] That day, different members of the group offered varied narratives and practices, addressing what was an appropriate way to behave in response to such brutal histories. However, as

---

2. For more discussion on the negotiation of Garifuna identity in New York City, see Oro (2020).

3. For a discussion of historical trauma among Native populations and an investigation into the "culture as treatment" model, see Gone (2013).

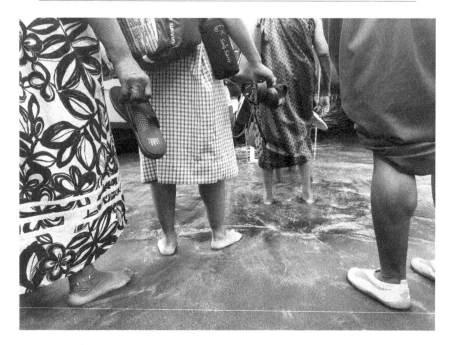

FIGURE 10 The Garifuna contingent from New York and Los Angeles boards the boat to Balliceaux, Yurumein (St. Vincent). Kristina Baines.

we came together on the rocky shore to drum and dance, to make tributes to the ancestors with candles and prayers, the collective experience offered both a space for celebration and for mourning. In the moments where conversation stopped and practice began, all, it seemed, were Garifuna first.

MUSIC AND THE COLLECTIVE MEMORY

"They are not coming here to fish. They are home attendants, teachers, train operators, military pilots, flight attendants, doctors, actors. Many will pass as Black American; they don't speak the language, and they don't care." Rosita's cousin, famed Garifuna musician James Lovell, was sitting in a Brooklyn bookshop, but he was speaking more broadly about the Belizean Garifuna diaspora in the United States. At the time of our conversation in 2017, his critique made sense. After several years of research,

I am not sure I agree with it in its entirety. I have met many Garifuna youth who speak the language, many more who care. And I have also met some fishers, who catch their fish in eastern Brooklyn and Queens and supply the ladies making hudut in the homes and churches of Bedford-Stuyvesant.

"When you come to the US, you are engaged in everything to survive, you acculturate, you assimilate, but the Garifuna is in you . . . it was in me; what drove me to myself was a love of music," James continued. He told me about how his people have a powerful history, and that he teaches youth to connect with this history and let people know that they will fight to keep it alive. He explained how he teaches them the names and purposes of traditional plants in nursery rhymes and children's songs. The songs often use familiar tunes and beats but are lyrically rich with Garifuna history and cultural knowledge. He continued, "I believe in social justice. I believe music can expose discrepancies; it can enlighten the masses." His explanation of collective memory resonates with scholarship on how music can create a collective sensation, an activation, or bubbling up, of pleasure and happiness, of ideas and memories.[4] He was activating the Garifuna inside the children he was working with and the members of the community who watched him perform. His discussion of his experiences was cast in quintessentially biocultural language. The distinct cultural practice, in this case Garifuna music, acts upon an internal physical body by way of a sensory experience, creating the awakening, the change in the way one feels. One feels more Garifuna, and that feeling of identity feels good.

"*Kasan buidubei Lun buidu Lan Basandiragun bunguwa.*" He teaches me how to ask what it takes to be healthy in Garifuna, and it is clear than my Garifuna has a long way to go before it rolls of the tongue in the same way as in Mopan Maya. He

---

4. This is a vast field of study. For a discussion of Durkheim's concept of collective effervescence in the context of collective emotions, see Collins (2014), and for an updated empirical study testing the concept, see Rimé and Páez (2023). Additionally, see Hsu (2022) for a discussion of the concept, as it relates to traditional medicinal and therapeutic techniques.

answers the question with a long list: peace of mind, no worries, no pain, feeling good in the body, well fed, comfortable, bills paid, children okay, me and my wife on good terms, loving toward each other. Although he had described his connection to music and Garifuna culture in this listing, he separated out "mind" and "body," illustrating how challenging it can be to marry the Garifuna worldview with the mind/body dualism that is pervasive in the United States.

Not too long after this meeting, I was introduced to Lisa, or Cookie, Rosita's niece, who also held Garifuna music classes for youth. We met at a Mexican restaurant in Los Angeles on a sunny afternoon and made our way through several baskets of tortilla chips as she explained to me how her priority is to connect her community to their culture, but, in Los Angeles, it was hard to maintain focus through the distractions. She had assumed many practices were common knowledge but had found out they are not. She understood why her community members were not always engaged with their Garifuna heritage but explained why she works to encourage her community to know and celebrate who they are. "Culture is your foundation; it explains your work ethic, your food choice . . ." We dipped our chips in the deliciously fresh salsa as she went on to share how celebrating the ancestors helps the Garifuna community develop as a people: "We are a cohesive people. I for you, you for me. These are our values." Garifuna values, of which collective care and respect for ancestors and their knowledge were most frequently discussed throughout my research encounters, she explained are not something that are explicitly talked about as values in some kind of external or abstract sense; they are enacted and reinforced every day. "Because of our heritage, we are able to make the decision [whether or not] we're going take the information and use it." She was offering music classes to the community and was also starting to offer cooking classes. "We use coconut milk here in LA, but fevergrass, they don't know what it's for. If you pick it up, they say, 'Where you from?'" She went on to explain that actually a lot of people do know what different medicinal plants are for, but they still "run for a bottle of aspirin." Knowledge is a critical first step, but it does not necessarily become practice. Cookie's description suggested that engaging with Garifuna culture was not simply an intellectual decision. Once one's body gets used to doing and eating in certain ways, it becomes a reflection of one's identity and values. People tap into their collective heritage identity through the memories that practice creates. Eating, dancing, and singing: these are all ways in which the body connects to the collective memory and the lived experience of heritage.

ANCESTRAL KNOWLEDGE, CALIFORNIA STYLE

"It was really something." Later that year, I was sitting around a polished dinner table in Long Beach, a smaller beachfront city west of Los Angeles, and a stylish woman in her fifties shared her experience learning to bake cassava bread in the traditional oven. She described the powerful sensation of the heat blowing on her face from the fire made in the brick construction built in her backyard. "Wow, this is what my ancestors did . . . this is mine," she explained as she described her experience, which she found, "liberating," "fun," and "deep." She described how she got the men to participate as well and people were still talking about it because it was so interactive. "Just the smell . . . it reminds me of home . . . the food feels like home . . . reminds me of my grandmother." Through her enthusiastic telling of her sensory experience—the heat on her skin, the smell evoking memories—it was clear that it was the experience rather than simply the knowledge that changed the way she thought about her heritage. She recognized that she would need to get members of her community *doing* and not just hearing about, watching, or even just eating the cassava bread. Her comment about the experience being interactive resonated. If participants did something, embodied a practice, rather than simply listened to a paper or watched a film, they would be more likely to talk about the experiences in other spaces as well, evoking the experience and generating interest in the practice or idea.[5] As she spoke, I felt the heat from the cassava bread baking in the brick oven.

"I love it; it's so 'rootsy'!" Her niece, also seated at the table, was discussing how she liked to participate in activities related to traditional Garifuna practice. Her cousin nodded and explained, "We need to eat our traditional foods; our ancestors ate organic." She went on to share how their elders lived a lot longer because they did not eat the processed food that is common both in Los Angeles and Belize these days. She told me about an initiative started by her family members who were creating vegan products inspired by traditional Garifuna flavors. They want to see their community move away from the fried foods common in current pan-Belizean cooking. Somehow this feels very California, with all its references related to clean eating and healthy living. It was not surprising that younger, Californian Garifuna communities emphasize the linear connection to biological health and longevity associated with vegetables, which feature prominently on the food pyramids taught in public school and other public health campaigns, even though these are not unique to California or the United States. However, as our multigenerational conversation unfolded, the picture that emerged at the table was more nuanced. The women spoke about healthy lives as woven into a collective experience, practices tied to projects and initiatives in classrooms and studios that differed from those one might find in kitchens and yards, but still involved coming together and embodying the ancestral knowledge to learn by *doing*.

MENTAL FOOD

I was walking quickly, the sandy pathways slowing my pace as I tried to keep up with the children leading me to my next destination. It was 2019 and my first time navigating around the sleepy Garifuna fishing village of Seine Bight on the Placencia

---

5. For more about embodied experience provoking conversation and memory see Baines and Costa (2022).

peninsula in the Stann Creek district of Belize. I had passed through the village many times on the way to visit friends, rest on the beach, and catch the snorkel boats to try and spot the ever-elusive whale sharks in Placencia village. My interest in Garifuna heritage practices now being known in the United States, I had been sent to find a relative, whose absence had sent me on to another. As I passed the familiar raised, wooden houses built high to avoid being swept away by the tides, I noticed several large concrete homes just paces away from the Caribbean Sea, brightly painted, with glossy, white shutters closed tight. The children eventually dipped back away from the shoreline and announced my presence to one of the local matriarchs, who listened to my tale of which relatives I knew in the United States with a mixture of skepticism and curiosity. Curiosity, with the addition of Garifuna hospitality, winning out, she invited me in to talk. "They pray; they are smart." We were talking about traditional Garifuna celebrations that take place in Seine Bight, what the ancestors demand at these events, and how those community members living away come back to take part. She was discussing mental health and the ancestors' critique of Western therapy—"We pray and sing and talk."

"Communities with a healthy social life have success and happiness." I nodded my head in agreement at the conclusion to this explanation of the challenges of maintaining healthy Garifuna communities in the United States. She explained the connection between contentment, food, culture, and tradition and said that living in the United States has killed the inner survival drive of the Garifuna people. In her view, Garifuna people in the United States have become more dependent on what has been manufactured for them, whether it be knowledge or food. She went on to describe Garifuna knowledge as "mental food," and her description aligned closely with the science of the proliferation of neurons in the gut, further entangling identity and the social, mental, and physical dimensions of health.[6]

---

6. For a discussion of the connection between mental health and the gut biome, see Järbrink-Sehgal and Andreasson (2020) and Bruce-Keller et al. (2018).

She handed me a Garifuna doll she had made and began to talk about the *dugu*, or ritual ceremony for the ancestors, which often brings families and the wider community together for several weeks. Some of her relatives were planning to come down from the United States for a dugu happening soon, and she had been preparing. She described the hanging of the clothes, the lighting of the candles, and the walking into the sea that would be part of the ceremony. I had heard a similar story a few months earlier from my Garifuna friends back in Los Angeles. They described how some family members were called back to Belize by the ancestors to participate in the dugu, but they could not travel due to the status of their immigration documents and, later, the 2020 COVID-19 pandemic restrictions. They decided to hold a version of the event in California, taking advantage of their proximity to the ocean. It was not as convenient as having a house right on the beach like in Seine Bight or Hopkins, but they managed to execute the critical pieces of the practice, the candles and the dyeing and hanging of the clothes. They had described how annatto was used to give the clothes their red color and how this also gave them a distinct smell. I was familiar with annatto, or achiote, a seasoning used by all ethnicities in Belize—a truly pan-Belizean spice. I knew it as *k'uxub* and had learned to process it back in southern Belize. Florentina, who taught me, was one of the last in Santa Cruz who still made k'uxub from scratch, although everyone still used it to make their caldo red, buying it from her or from other Maya ladies in the market.[7] I remembered her warning me that making it was hard, but it was not until the sharp spikes of the dried pods dug into my soft, stained fingers, damp from pulling the fleshy seeds from the inside that I realized why not many people extracted it. Garifuna community members certainly bought their annatto back in Los Angeles, staining the white cloth red to remember

---

7. Processing annatto for sale is seeing a resurgence of interest across Belize in recent years as part of a growing interest in developing small cottage industries around traditional and "natural" Belizean products, including coconut oil and cohune nut oils as other prominent examples.

the dead and honor the ancestors. As they evoked the sensations of the red clothes drying on the line, blowing in the breeze, dispersing the very faint smell of the annatto, I was grateful to hear about the process.

Similarly, I was pleasantly surprised to hear the details again as I sat here in Seine Bight. For much of Garifuna history, the dugu had been one of the ceremonies hidden from outsiders, likely out of a very real fear of persecution. Now, the dugu was emerging as an important way for the younger generation to reconnect with their Garifuna heritage, and with their ancestors. Furthermore, the ritual often brought younger Garifuna people from all over the United States back home. Later in the conversation. when I asked about all the empty houses on the beaches and if anyone would ever live there, she scolded, "Of course, they come back; this is their home."

NARRATIVES OF RETURN

"I want to talk to you. After breakfast." My eyes widened as I began to imagine what I had done wrong. Although I had been made to feel very welcome on this trip to St. Vincent, and I was thoroughly enjoying myself, I was still self-conscious about coming along on such an important homecoming trip to Yurumein and witnessing such an emotional ancestral reconnection. I must have shown disrespect, I thought. However, when I went to talk to Hazel after breakfast, her stern countenance quickly changed to a sly smile. "It's time to get your Garifuna clothes," she instructed. I understood this as her way of welcoming me into her inner circle, a signal of trust, and the beginning of a deepening of our friendship. Hazel was the only member of the NYC and LA communities that I had met who hailed from Barranco, the only Garifuna village in the Toledo district of Belize, a place known for being a center for Garifuna heritage. I had remembered the Maya leaders telling me that they felt the closest connection with the community in Barranco, in part because of its physical proximity to the Q'eqchi' villages in the south and, thus, similar ecological considerations, even though it was right on the sea. The communities in the Toledo district, or the "forgotten district" as it was often referred to, had also historically been the most removed from the development projects and processes and so were perhaps more tightly hewed to their heritage practices. Hazel and I shared knowing conversations about the particularities of the Toledo district, the slow pace of life, and the Indigenous values she found important. "Many hands make a light basket," she reminded me in one of those moments as I thought back to all the times when I had been told that the community coming together to help one another was critical to a healthy, happy life.

In the summer of 2023 at her apartment in Brooklyn, she offered an example to illustrate the connection between collective activities and being well, one she had experienced many times growing up in Barranco: "When you have the harvest of the cassava roots to make cassava bread, everyone comes to peel the cassava. They all come with their graters, the long boards, and grate the cassava. They'll be in their long skirts, grating and singing, giving it rhythm, then we put it in the *wowla* to drain it and get the poison out—this is the only time [during the process] that kids were welcome. We need them to sit on it to drain it! When you see people doing that task, everybody is happy because they are singing together and working together. The neighbors will come over without you asking them, and when it is finished, they get their piece [of cassava bread]." She continued to explain how she grew up in Maya communities in Belize because her parents were teachers. They could speak Q'eqchi' to the students, and they observed the same principle of coming together or working together in community—it was a Maya value just like it was a Garifuna value. She was visibly excited telling the story and then seemed slightly saddened. "It's not like before, and I don't know why." She offered a critique of life today, along with some thoughts about reasons why. "I keep telling young people to keep active—to go for a walk. Before we were going to the plantation, [harvesting] and processing by hand, and now a machine can do it. The comal used to be on the ground, and the stove is high now.

These changes are making everything easier, so you don't have to bend your body so you get fatter. We used to have to grate the coconuts with our parents. That was hard work!"

A few weeks earlier, I was sitting under the green house by the water tank in Dangriga learning about the hard work expected of the earlier generations of Garifuna. We had gathered here after the celebratory mass to mark one year since Marciana's passing. Her children and grandchildren had come from the United States, and friends and neighbors came by to talk about her life while enjoying *bimecacule*, or sweet rice, and other nourishments common at gatherings to remember and honor those who had passed away. Laughter erupted as Marciana's daughter told the story of processing sorrel when they were young. She detailed how their fingers would be raw from the moisture and the prickles, and I thought back to the Maya achiote processing I had come to know with my own hands. She touched her fingers, remembering that feeling as she recalled how her mother tasked her with the job. Remembering their mother that day for her children, now the older generation, meant remembering the sensations of their childhood work. They, too, recalled the processing of coconut and cassava, explaining that helping with this hard work was not presented to them as an option. They learned it, they did it, and they remembered it with their bodies. And through remembering it, back in the place of their childhood, they remembered her. Her grandchildren present at the event, two of Rosita's daughters who had traveled from the United States, shared with me how they keep Garifuna traditions, cooking traditional foods. They organized a family outing after the gathering had come to a close to visit Hopkins and eat some hudut. Excited to be invited to join, I was struck by how this was the first time I had been asked how I wanted my soup: with fish, lobster, pigtail, white or brown gravy. Tailoring their traditional meal to their individual tastes was a way of engaging with heritage practices on their own terms, choice being a part of everyday American culture. Marciana's extended family gathering together and eating this meal in the stiff sea breeze exemplified how the now-middle generation engaged with their heritage practices in a very considered and visible way. They confidently embodied the "best of both worlds" model in response to changing dynamics and locations.

Hazel knew I was going to visit Belize soon after we returned from Yurumein in 2019, and she encouraged me to go see her house and visit her son, who had recently opened one of the only restaurants in Barranco. When we met, a few months later, sitting in his restaurant refueling with a cold drink after the long and muddy drive down the notoriously rough, unpaved road from Punta Gorda, he explained that the community was planning an event for the next summer. There would be a dugu and a celebration of Garifuna culture and practice, and the young people in the diaspora would be returning to come together and build community. He wanted to reinvigorate and reimagine his community through engagement with his home and his culture. The young people had no way to connect to their ancestors, and he and others wanted to get to know their relatives who lived far away. The next summer the airport to Belize closed because of the COVID-19 pandemic, so there was no traveling to Belize for younger Garifuna people living in the United States, and so there was no event.

Despite this, young Garifuna adults did not abandon their desire to embrace their heritage. Unable to travel to Belize, they turned to Facebook groups and virtual conferences to reconnect with Garifuna heritage.[8] There was a narrative emerging on social media and in these conferences that the youth should move back to Barranco, but some of those in the conversation had to answer to some criticism from others living further north and in the diaspora: "Why are you regressing like that." The narratives of return to place, to heritage practices, were made visible through social media; however, an online conference, I was told, can both minimize and overstate the transformation taking place among the Garifuna community. "It's a movement," one

---

8. The practice of diasporic communities using social media to connect with family and culture is well documented. See Komito (2011) and González and Castro (2007).

self-proclaimed activist stressed. "Long before the internet, we had the conch shell and the coconut wireless." The now-older generation seems cautious when considering these new, visible heritage movements. They have questioned the motivations of those who have newly rediscovered their heritage practice. Deep knowledge and understanding needs to precede practice, the elders stress, especially when making money is involved.

Commodification, especially of heritage practices such as the dugu, is looked upon with a skeptical eye. Hazel offered some advice for young people based on her own experience: "They should go back and stay there and get a piece of land. There are many empty pieces of land in Barranco. Go back there. Everybody has different values, but one thing my father always preached about, 'Don't forget where you came from.'" When she moved to the United States, she told me, he made her promise to build her house in Barranco, because her children love to go there. So she did. And they do. Her comments encapsulated a common sentiment: even if you are *lisurnia*, you will always be Baranguna.[9]

Back in California, Lisa "Cookie" was explaining how everyone needs to go back to Belize to maintain the connection. Returning to Belize was often mentioned as essential to both a restoration of health and of Garifuna values, which themselves are explicitly intertwined. In Belize, she continued, "you can be very rich [or poor] and buy your fruit at the same fruit stand." Cookie was contrasting life in Belize with what she was casting as the individualistic mindset that goes hand in hand with the economic disparities she saw playing out in California. When members of the diaspora return to Belize, they are clearly wealthier than those in their home communities, as evidenced by the shuttered concrete houses in Seine Bight—and in nearly every town or village in Belize. However, she made the point that eating the same fruit bought from the same fruit stand will actually restore their Garifunaness

---

9. According to Palacio, Lumb, and Tuttle (2009), *lisurnia* is a Garifuna word, meaning "away from one's home community for a period of lime" with the understanding that you will return home. Baranguna refers to "one who belongs to Barranco."

and keep them well regardless of their economic standing. I had heard similar talk of the return to Belize in Brooklyn—people had talked about wanting to go back to fish, to go to the river to wash clothes, "to find something of home." Those practices that cannot be replicated can perhaps be restored, the body recharged and repaired through this reconnection.

I met Alice on the homecoming trip to Yurumein in 2019, and she invited me to visit her at her home in Los Angeles early the next year. I met her at a park near the Belizean Garifuna community in South Central Los Angeles, taking a walk before we returned to her home and, much to my excitement, made panades with fish for lunch. She liked to make sure she got her exercise, as many in the community were getting diabetes and high blood pressure. As we slowly rounded the small running track multiple times, she talked about her childhood in Seine Bight and what she had learned since she had been in Los Angeles and made return trips back to her village. When she was last in Seine Bight a few years earlier, she experienced a pain in her knee, and a man said to peel the green mango and take the skin, boil it, and drink it. She also learned to drink the *nehu* or okra water. "Stuff like that the kids need to know, somebody needs to tell them," she told me. She confided to me that her father would not let her go to the Garifuna cultural events in Seine Bight when she was growing up there, that he would not let her and her siblings take part in the dancing. I wondered aloud if this was motivated by fear or perhaps by her father's Christian religion. She did not speculate but said she learned more about the Garifuna culture in Los Angeles than she did growing up in Belize. When I asked her how Garifuna children might learn these things, the dancing, the language, the traditional medicinal therapies, she suggested that the community produce pictures with words in Garifuna for children to take home and put on the wall. She also suggested making ground food for lunches, so children could get used to the traditional foods.[10] I nodded,

---

10. "Ground food" is a classification of locally grown tubers such as cassava and yams and, often, different banana species that is used across

having noticed the rough brown tubers of cassava at the grocery store in the neighborhood when I stopped to pick up some fruit to contribute to our lunch. They were there surrounded by aisles of sodas and endcaps of packaged cakes and cookies, a well-documented phenomenon, particularly in less-wealthy neighborhoods.[11] Through my fieldwork experiences augmented by having married into a Cuban family, I knew how much time and effort went into processing cassava, or yuca as they called it. When I imagined kids growing up in South Central Los Angeles, swinging by the grocery store, there was little wonder why Alice pointed to the need for a very focused effort to bring these foods to the youth. The older people needed them too, with the rising rates of chronic disease we had discussed earlier, a phenomenon on everyone's mind. For Alice and other Garifuna living in Los Angeles, the traditional ways were better, fresher, and more nourishing, but it continued to be a struggle to incorporate them into daily lives here.

KNOW YOUR HISTORY AND TAKE CARE OF YOUR BODY

I met Nickey, Cookie's cousin, in Los Angeles a few times, but we were just getting to know each other when the 2020 pandemic pause came into effect. She was active in the community and a powerful organizer, also keen to share her personal stories as a way to demonstrate how someone could live their heritage in a place like Los Angeles. We were connected on social media, and I began to notice posts she shared related to the promotion of Garifuna heritage, which intrigued me in terms of their diversity. Remembering the genocide on Balliceaux, which is often

---

ethnicities in Belize and is a popular example of a type of healthy food.

11. Structural inequities in the availability of fresh food versus processed food in poorer neighborhoods in the United States is well documented but persists. See Reese (2018) for a discussion of food access and health consequences in the frame of racial and economic disadvantage.

glossed over in Garifuna histories, was gaining critical importance in the community, with images and detailed text, dates, and drawings being shared.[12] I read these with eager curiosity, our return trip to Yurumein having been put on hold during the pandemic. In large text at the bottom of one of the posts, which consisted of several maps and quotes from colonial texts, I read, "Every Garifuna Had a Least 4 Ancestors In the 1797 Garifuna Exile Genocide Attempt 2 Maternal Ancestors and 2 Paternal Ancestors."[13] Garifuna community members were appealing to Garifuna both in Belize and in the diaspora, reminding them that they had a personal connection to the devastating colonial histories and a responsibility to honor the ancestors through understanding and keeping up with their Garifuna cultural identity. Knowledge was critical, and it perhaps was the key to practice.

A return to in-person gatherings was marked on social media with a flyer advertising "Garifunarobics!," an exercise class with live drumming. This flyer reminded me about the Garifuna chefs who were preparing vegan food: traditional foodways, California style. This class had traditional music, California style. Both classes targeted a Western biomedical narrative of a healthy lifestyle, which included healthy diet and exercise, while incorporating the traditional practices known to intersect with the experience of being Garifuna in the world. These seemed a clear expression of syncretic, or blended, health behavior well-documented and discussed in Garifuna communities.[14] The need for a biomedical approach to health seemed critical, as

---

12. Both scholarly and popular accounts of the Garifuna exile to Balliceaux by the British colonizers, which resulted in the deaths of over two thousand Garifuna people, have increased in visibility over the past decade. See Finneran and Welch (2020) and Joseph (2020) for more on the role of the history of Balliceaux in Garifuna collective memory.

13. From 1797 Garifuna Exile, Quick Reference Guide, Joycelin Palacio-Cayetano, PhD (series of Facebook posts).

14. For an account of therapeutic syncretism in a Garifuna community, see Staiano (2016, 65).

chronic disease, notably diabetes (or "sugar" or "sweet blood") and hypertension (or "pressure") seemed to be on everyone's mind. Their mental health was also affected as a result, or as part of a circular process of declining health. Stress, or "worries," was discussed in both Garifuna and Maya communities. Some of this stress, and overall sickness, seemed to be related to changes: food was more expensive, harder to get reliably since the pandemic. Lifestyles had changed. People were busy working for money and did not have the long hours available to process cassava or corn. This lack of time increased the need for more money to buy more expensive and already processed food. A reliance on this food led to more chronic disease. What Nickey and others have shown is that heritage practice might go some distance to interrupt this process. Rather than Indigenous communities being defined by poor health and their indigeneity somehow being synonymous with this, they are finding ways that their indigeneity can be and is protective and health-promoting. The increasing visibility of alternative practices might have real consequences for health outcomes—and for healthy Indigenous futures.

CHAPTER 6

TOWARD A SENSORY ECOLOGY OF THERAPEUTICS

IT TOOK JUST FORTY MINUTES to reach the Santa Cruz village now, a decade later, with buses running along the new road from Punta Gorda, or Peini, as the new colorful sign reminds us is the town's Garifuna name. They hurtle down to Jalacte at the Guatemala border and back again with a frequency that is still jarring to me. The bus journey, once an arduous several hours' ride along a pitted, muddy stretch of the highway, was now quick and easy, allowing for frequent daily rides in and out of town, if a person could afford the fare. Flows of people, goods, and cattle moved back and forth along the road, and the planning and discussions of when people would go into town next became increasingly obsolete. Going to high school became easier, the trip shorter and school closer than it had ever been. People were traveling to cross into Guatemala just to "take a walk around." Since the 2020–2021 pandemic closed the borders to migrant farm workers from elsewhere in Central America, buses were sent into Santa Cruz and neighboring villages early in the morning to pick up people to work in the banana farms up on the Southern Highway, the paved road bringing them back again every evening. On my most recent trip, it was tough to find who I was looking for at home, when before it had been easy. It was a good thing it was no longer challenging to come back the next day.

As expected, the road had brought changes.[1] Some were significant—and the pandemic restrictions amplified these. It was easy to find examples of the impacts of the paving of roads on community health. Paved roads are linked to an increase in chronic disease, with processed foods making their way into communities with more ease.[2] Just as in Garifuna communities in Los Angeles, more Maya people here talked about "sweet blood," but it was unclear if many more people actually had diabetes or the ease of clinic visits had made a medical diagnosis more likely. Paved roads also made working for cash outside the villages easier. Ease of travel to high school, in turn, increased the pressure to work for that cash to pay for school fees and meals away from home.

As I climbed onto the bus and rode out of Santa Cruz village for one last time, the driver nodded:

"Hi, Kristina. So, you're back again?"

"Yes, how is everything?"

"Well, the same."

As the bus rounded the corners and dropped down the hills on the way to join the Southern Highway, only a small change in the velocity of the wind on my face indicated a change in the road surface. The view, layers of lush forest, wide-leaved lau, and traveler palms spread out across the landscape, punctuated by towering cohune palms, remained remarkably similar. As the bush gave way to roadside shops in the passing villages, I noticed some had gone out of business, while others seem to have expanded. Solar panels brought more ice-cold drinks to

---

1. For a discussion of the expectations related to the paving of this road, see Haines (2018).

2. For a detailed discussion of the effects of "modernity" on the health of Indigenous populations, see Wiedman (2012). For a discussion of related diabetes drivers, and heritage practices as resilience, in Maya communities in southern Belize, see Schmidt (2022).

buy. In very little time, we were already rounding the corner at the Caribbean Sea, where a couple of kids were swimming off a wooden dock. The water was flat like glass, disturbed only by the children. The fishing boats were tied for the evening. The pandemic pause and the unrelenting sea breeze had left many spots in need of a fresh coat of paint. Maybe they had always needed that fresh coat of paint. How changed was this place really?

I got off the bus and smiled at a young woman I had come to know. She was cooking in the small kitchen off to the side of the shop by the bus stop, and I hoped that she still had some fish for me to eat with my rice and beans.

"Thank you; I will see you next time."
"Yes, next time. If we are still alive."
"Yes, if we are still alive."

CONCLUSIONS AND BEGINNINGS

Through the gathering of these stories, I was changed. My notebooks were full, but I had indeed learned with my body. Through the sharing of these stories, I have aimed to honor that learning in both celebration and critique. By way of both summary and introduction to these concluding thoughts, this is what Belizean Maya and Garifuna communities living in times of change (which is always) have taught me:

- Tradition is not static or archaic but nuanced and negotiated, embodied and lived in the everyday.
- Traditional practice is not a rejection of change or of modernity.
- "Traditional" is a word used by communities to describe a wide range of practices, and, as such, it is a useful classificatory tool.
- Traditional practices are linked to health.
- Health is holistic.

- Assumptions about traditional healing systems and their clashes with science or biomedical models contain false dichotomies.

And this is what I have learned from these lessons:

- Phenomenological perspectives and sensory experiences can be scientifically understood, even if we are still honing the tools to measure them.
- Sensory experiences act upon the physical body.
- The mind is part of the body.
- The body is part of the community and the entire ecological system.
- Inherent in this argument is a critique of biomedicine and biopower but not a rejection of it.
- Inherent in the argument is a critique of global development thinking, which privileges biomedicine and other associated ways of being in the world as more aspirational and more valid than others.
- Inherent in this argument is an economic critique, a critique of capital, of the resultant health disparities, of hyperindividualism, and of the supremacy of individual bodies.
- Traditional practice often means collective practice.
- Community-focused therapeutic practice can go some distance to heal collective trauma associated with being Indigenous, with being marginalized, with being colonized, with the ongoing challenging and dismissal of your belief systems.

Foremost, I have learned that change is hard but that life continues in ways that are rich and beautiful. The stories I have gathered here are not simply a critique of global forces or hegemonic systems: they are also a celebration of the joys and discoveries of daily life in the midst of inevitable and ongoing changes.

DO YOUR TRADITIONS

"How can we keep our traditions when the government is selling it?" I was waiting at the bus stop in Punta Gorda and struck up a conversation in rusty Mopan with a fellow traveler, a lean, middle-aged Maya man with a wide smile. We did not start talking about traditions, but, after a few minutes of chitchat, which included speculation as to when the bus would arrive and which village everyone was headed to, we exchanged names. "Are you the Kristina who wrote that book? I read that. That was a good book!" I nodded, trying to contain my excitement at the revelation that he both read the book and thought it was good. He then quickly went on to explain how he agreed with the community members I had spoken to, and with the conclusions of my research. Traditions really were important, but he explained that it was getting increasingly more difficult to practice them these days. He sat on a plastic armchair outside a cement block shop. I asked if I could take a photo to document our meeting. His smiling face was framed by the advertisements for the newest brand of imported energy drink sold inside. I thought about how many times I had been served cacao drink after long mornings of working to prepare food for those planting corn or building houses, and thought to myself: *Cacao: the original energy drink, since 1500 BC!* I was just starting to encounter cacao ceremonies making their way to New Age enclaves in the United States, which left me uncomfortable despite my understandings of how knowledge and practice flow through time and space. Perhaps my discomfort was related to my new friend's opening statement about the commodification of traditions and traditional practice by others in positions of power. I took his governmental critique to have several layers. The relationship between land, natural resources, and traditional practice is clear, particularly in the Toledo district, and the role of government in claiming and selling Indigenous lands is, unfortunately, an old story.[3] While Maya communities have

---

3. As an example, for a discussion of the history of Indigenous disenfranchisement in Guatemala, in addition to a recent discussion of how

claimed their land rights and the government has acknowledged them, they have yet to be fully codified, and communities continue to struggle to maintain their land management practices amid various pushbacks, both subtle and overt. His statement also encapsulated the way the Belizean government, in his view, has historically packaged and sold Maya cultural heritage identity, notably in the form of pictures of ancient Mayan pyramids on their tourist brochures and websites. Maya culture is essentially frozen in time and commodified for the gain of government-sanctioned private tour operators, most of whom are not Maya themselves. In the case of cacao specifically, the commodification is not limited to foreigners. Local, family-run chocolate-making ventures have increased throughout southern Belize to capitalize on the ever-growing visibility of the origins of the sweet treat in the cacao tree. Tourists take chocolate tours, roasting cacao seeds and grinding them with the mano and metate, the heavy stones a testament perhaps to the continued strength of Maya people.

Reimagining traditions in a community-led capitalist frame is one way in which they persist. Like the marimba demonstrations along the Southern Highway or the Garifunarobics classes, cacao demonstrations make cultural practices visible to outsiders, but also to youth in the communities. There are problematics to consider. There are risks associated with essentializing culture for noncritical consumption: encouraging tourists to see communities as quaint relics of collapsed civilizations, freezing them in time. The relevance of Indigenous knowledge and practice in the twenty-first century is both strengthened and weakened through these kinds of revivals and demonstrations. These sorts of cultural projects are not explicitly and uncritically about "saving Indigenous knowledge," although that is how they might be framed in the context of funding agencies and other external supports. However, the commodification of traditions allows their practice to be prioritized over working for cash in other ways, for commercial enterprises like in construction or

---

this has been linked to addressing health inequities, see Hernandez et al. (2022).

administration or hospitality. There is some evidence that these projects aimed at visibility and promotion of traditional practice serve a role in offering prestige and value to the younger generation.[4] The common narrative that traditional practices are lost as the trappings of modernity increase, while not without evidence, lacks detail and the understandings that the practices persist, even in the wake of global capitalism.[5] Pressures of the market economy, and porous social structures that result from the hyperindividualism of capitalist engagement, are perceived to erode Indigenous practice and debase Indigenous knowledge; however, these same pressures, when acted upon with intentionality, can intensify these practices. I have learned that, in the Belizean Indigenous context, health is a mitigating factor in this seemingly complex and contradictory relationship. Simply stated, the pressures of this capitalist engagement are associated with negative health outcomes, and the traditional practices are associated with positive ones. When you embody your ecological heritage, you are more well.

In discussions of EEH, I use the term "ecological" in a broad, systemic sense to place individual bodily practices in the context of wider ecologies, reinforcing how those connections inform people's lived experience. "Ecological" is often colloquially used as synonymous with "environmental," and although I chose to use it for its systemic meaning, Indigenous heritage practices are often quite explicitly connected to the land or environmental materials—for example, rivers and plants.[6] I found this with frequency among both the Maya and Garifuna communities. The

---

4. See the documentary film *The Last Bonesetter* (Booher and Oths 2018) for an account of how the practice of a Peruvian healer was captured and formalized in order to garner the interest of youth in the community.

5. For an example, see the discussion of the practice of shamanism still found in Nepal during Maoist revolutions in Zharkevich (2019).

6. For discussions of the relationship between natural elements and Indigenous knowledge and practice, see Kimmerer (2020) and Black Elk (2016).

pandemic was coming to its official end in 2022 when I started to get pinged on Facebook messenger with YouTube links with titles such as "How we potentiate fruit bearing trees: a brief look at Garifuna Ceremonial Agriculture" and "Messages of Natural Health for the Diaspora, Caribbean." These came from Arzu Mountain Spirit, whom I had always known as Doctor Arzu, a Garifuna Belizean American healer whom I had met in Punta Gorda many years prior. Combining knowledge of her medical school training in New York City and her ancestral ethnobotanical and ritual practice, she had provided therapeutic treatments to a wide range of Toledo residents and visitors. In her videos, she walked around her garden, sharing some contemplative moments with the plants she had growing there. The way in which you interacted with the plants, she showed us, was just as important as the healing chemicals in the plants. Thinking back to the Maya healers' desire to legitimize their practice within the growing biomedical context of Belize—the "scientific verification" of botanical healing practices—I wondered if she had ever been called upon to do this. When I paid her a postpandemic visit to catch up, I was able to ask her about her series. She told me, "My goal was to put the plant spirituality of our people on the map because I knew we had something special. Everybody has access. I have the right to have access to my parents—the earth is my mother—everyone has the right to the medicines the earth grows. They are for all of us." She has had many encounters with scientific verification processes but rejects the frame that supports the exclusivity and hyperprofessionalization of traditional plant knowledge.

Doctor Arzu's face, both on her videos and in person, seemed to illuminate when she was sharing what she described as her ancestral knowledge. She touched the plants and their fruits carefully, slowly taking a moment to experience what they shared with her. The physicality of walking through her space, the materiality of the soft leaves, the rough bark, a ripeness of the fruits to the touch, the smell of the blossoms, and the damp soil—all these momentary practices seemed to build into a kind of "sensory nostalgia," a connection with the rich joys of remembering through practice.[7] The plants, through their olfactory engagement with those caring for them, provided a connection to homelands, reminders of how displacement and disenfranchisement might be mitigated through the sensory. I was learning that smells travel across time and space with bodies, captured as memories through sensory experiences, and interactions between them can be activated to evoke the ecological connections, even after long periods of time being dormant. Studies show people experience an increased sense of well-being in gardens, and the sparkle in Doctor Arzu's eyes told me she felt healthier too—mind, body, and soul.[8]

THE SCIENCE OF THE SENSORY

Before we even got to the bridge, we could see the plumes of thick white smoke rising from behind the trees alongside the river. As we reached the middle of the bridge, we hollered down to the ladies in the river below. They looked up with smiles and waved, returning to their work cleaning the lengths of smooth, creamy-colored pig intestines in the gently moving water. We continued walking and began to smell the smoke wafting on the breeze—the unmistakably rich, delicious smell of roasting pork. As we turned off the bridge, we wandered through the space between the houses, one made of cement blocks with a zinc

---

7. Biglin (2020) used the term "sensory nostalgia" when she was making sense of her observations of refugees in an urban community garden in the United Kingdom. Smelling the basil they had planted there, she argued, was an inherently political act.

8. Discussion of the many articulations and conceptions of the soul worldwide is beyond the scope of this book; however, it is included here because of the way in which it was discussed by Doctor Arzu in the context of holistic health. Other Belizean community members did not regularly use this term, although there was often a generalized supernatural component to discussions of holistic health.

roof and one made of a more traditional thatch and board, to the backyard, where large slabs of meat were resting on a large makeshift grill made of thick sticks, with the glowing embers of a sprawling fire underneath. Eluterio approached, a slow, slight

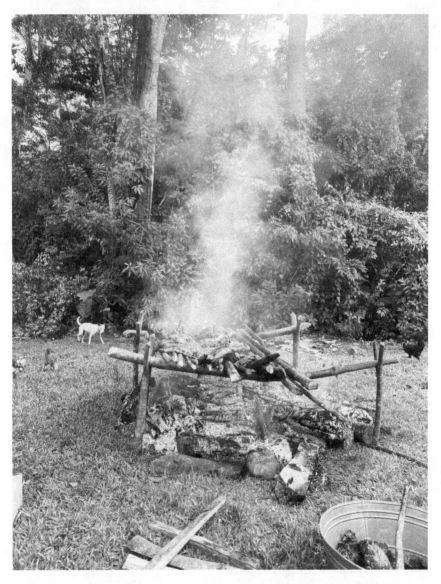

FIGURE 11 Pig roasting for the birthday gathering, Santa Cruz village, Toledo, Belize. Kristina Baines.

irregularity in his gait, and we wished him a happy birthday as he informed us that he killed two pigs for his celebration and that one of them was over four hundred pounds. He was a well-known village elder and pastor in the Baptist church and had a lot of people to feed. He shared that he was roasting the meat because it removes a lot of the fat. Too much fat and sugar, he explained, are not good for your health. I had known about his struggle with diabetes, and, the next day, after our caldo and cake, he told me that he had lost his foot to the disease. This was the first amputation due to diabetic neuropathy I had heard about in a Maya community in Toledo, although I knew they had been increasing in Garifuna communities at alarming rates in recent years.[9] The relationship between modernity and chronic disease is well-documented, and it was no surprise that Eluterio had been one of the first people in the village to own a vehicle and to have a shop. Even since he had first shown signs of illness, his narratives about the relationships between a movement away from traditional practice and declining health had been clear.[10] This celebration of his life with a traditional meal, punctuated by a deliciously sugary cake of which he did not partake, highlights the multiplicity of ways in which the social and cultural become embodied in the metabolic system.

The nature/culture argument, when considering human health behaviors and outcomes, is one that is both overemphasized and underproblematized. Like many epistemological dichotomies, it crystallizes ways of thinking around operational pieces of information on which programs and projects are based. This serves to reinforce a kind of scientific arrogance that can be damaging to those navigating their paths to the maintenance of health. Focusing on the body, and the way it moves through the world, moves consideration beyond this separation of nature and culture and toward an understanding that the world is not what people think

---

9. See Moran-Thomas (2019) for a detailed account of diabetes among the Garifuna communities in Belize.

10. See chap. 3 of Baines (2016a), "Embodying Ecological Heritage in a Maya Community," for Eluterio's account of his diabetes onset.

but what they live.[11] This phenomenological approach is central to the argument for a sensorial and embodied understanding of how health is constructed and maintained. Emerging with clarity from the ethnographies of everyday Indigenous Belizeans in an ever-changing world, narratives of sensory experience are rich in the convergence of the biological and the cultural in the body, demonstrating how sensations are "experienced phenomenologically, interpreted culturally, and responded to socially.[12]" "Local phenomenologies" can be described as "constituted by both local analytic theories of experience and lived experience itself and assumes these influence one another to some degree."[13] For example, when a Garifuna grandmother in Brooklyn rubs the flesh of a lime on the body to cool it, this cools the body through its moisture and chemical composition (citric acid), while the smell of the tart flesh and sensation on the skin are experienced as a cooling practice. Her grandchild might both experience the sensation and think about the sensation as one associated with feeling better. The lime might also serve as a conduit for the grandmother's touch and care. Limes as cooling—keeping Garifuna well in the health of both the Belizean and the Brooklyn summer—are understood as such through physical, material factors converging with the social in the body.

Phenomenological explanations for health and healing modalities are not new. From philosophers to physiologists, thinking about the lived experience, mitigated by the senses, has proven fruitful to better understand how people find their place in the world. Yet, despite this high-profile work, I still find myself challenged—by scholars, health professionals, students, and friends—to demonstrate how the cultural becomes biological

---

11. There is a robust literature engaging the nature/culture dichotomy. For a detailed call for moving beyond the nature/culture dichotomy from anthropology, see Fassin (2007). For other perspectives on this dualism, see Haila (2000) and Descola (2006).

12. For detailed discussions of what is termed "sensorial anthropology," see Nichter (2008).

13. See Halliburton (2002).

when I make the case for the links between practice and identity and health.[14] It is helpful, perhaps, to return to the example of the lime and investigate what I will call the mechanism of sensory therapeutics. Underneath the skin, physiologists have isolated tiny sensors called vesicles or exosomes, which experience sensations and transmit these to the brain. This may not seem like a revelation; however, the critical piece is how these vesicles connect with other organs of the body, the brain being just one of many, and how this process creates a therapeutic space within it.

Embodied ecological heritage as a framework incorporates a cognitive perspective within phenomenological experience, rather than standing in opposition to it. I consider several factors to clarify this relationship between cognition and phenomenology: "what is initially embodied and sensorial may, over time, *become cognitive* as narrative; explanation and meaning become attached to the experience."[15] This goes some distance to explaining, for example, how feeling the lime on one's skin when one is young can lead to discussing it as a healing practice; however, I ask if this goes far enough. If we press harder against the Cartesian separation of mind and body, the changes in ways of thinking around the lime are the result of the activation of the vesicles in the nostrils, the saliva, the skin, and their connection to the brain through the neurophysiological system. And this neurophysiological physiological system is linked to the genetic system. So, when the Garifuna and Maya talk about hudut or caldo as being part of their DNA, they are making an epigenetic argument, connecting the needs of their biology to the needs of their culture through practice. Fulfilling those needs is part of leading a healthy life.

But are they actually healthier? I feel as though I have become accustomed to answering versions of this question in various

---

14. For a physiological perspective, see Noble (2022). For an updated discussion of the "biocultural synthesis," see Leatherman and Goodman (2020). For an understanding of the relationships between sociocultural phenomena and biological change, see Dressler et al. (2005).

15. For a discussion of how the phenomenological becomes cognitive, see Thompson, Ritenbaugh, and Nichter (2009) and Ingold (2020).

kinds of spaces for decades, even using it as a title for a recent article.[16] Anthropologists (medical anthropologists, in particular) have long made the case that belief systems (in this case, health belief systems) have foundations in different systems of truth.[17] Bioscience is one of those systems. The dichotomy between what is a belief and what is a scientific fact reflects the same kind of scientific arrogance I am hoping to address through these stories. The body is both "soft evidence" and "hard evidence." Maya and Garifuna experiences of embodied health support a call for humility in regards to the natural system. They go some distance to combat the narrative of the primacy of Western scientific practice as producing the only "hard evidence." To devalue or ignore the material changes observed through traditional healing practice creates an "epistemic injustice" or acts as a kind of "bio-epistemicide" of Indigenous ways of thinking.[18] This is a powerful critique, one which my learning documented in the stories in this book supports. However, with these stories of Indigenous communities living in times of change, I aim to think *with* Western science and not against it. These Indigenous sensory experiences and connections of being and living in the world are science and their practitioners, scientists.[19]

Philosophers argue that even science has a metaphysical position.[20] I am always thinking back to the ongoing damage of Des-

---

16. Baines (2018).

17. See Fassin (2007, 122).

18. Gebara (2023) elaborated on this critique at the Green Templeton College Conference for Human Welfare.

19. Indigenous communities are scientists in the sense that they draw conclusions through observations of the natural world. Aspects of Western scientific methodology—replicability and controlled environments as examples—may not be employed by the community members represented in this statement.

20. Science and Technology Studies (STS) deals directly with questions of the ideology behind science as empirical truth set against the field of science being firmly rooted in its own set of Eurocentric values and practices. For an overview of the development of STS, see Fuller and Collier (2003). Sjöstedt-Hughes (2023) elaborated on this observation from an

cartes's legacy. His successful call for separation of the mind from the body in Western thought not only disenfranchised other species, whose intelligence has shown to be remarkable across so many studies, but has also become embedded the primacy of Western scientific thought into what would become biomedical training.[21] In the project of unraveling and addressing the racist and colonial histories, "taking seriously embodied ways of knowing" goes some distance to trusting what communities tell us about their bodies and their health.[22]

DEVELOP TO WHERE?

Our bodies were sweating in the trapped afternoon heat, vibrating with the kinetic sound of the fat, tropical raindrops landing on the zinc roof. We could feel their velocity and frequency bouncing around—roof, bodies, walls . . . We sat in the Santa Cruz community center, where I had been invited to a meeting to talk about some development projects that were ongoing in the village, and some that needed to be discussed and interest gauged before they might be accepted. Gathering the community for the purpose of sharing information and engaging in collective decision-making is a traditional practice in Maya communities in southern Belize. The *ab'ink*, or listening session, serves practical purposes but also reinforces Maya values related to collectivity and community-led practice. As the community leaders presented the information, I found myself straining to hear. This was not the first time I had experienced frustration

---

explicitly philosophical perspective at the Green Templeton College Conference for Human Welfare.

21. Intelligence and agency in nonhuman beings has been demonstrated notably by Narby (2005), Kirksey and Helmreich (2010), and Tsing (2013).

22. Garth (2023) discusses how her research supports the validity of embodied ways of knowing, drawing from Thomas's 2019 employment of Black feminist critique of colonial knowledge holders.

during an afternoon rainstorm, and it was commonly known that zinc roofs amplified the sound of these common occurrences during the rainy season. We took short breaks when the sound intensified to impossible levels, and pressed on when possible, the cement block building holding in the heat as temperatures and tensions rose. In the end, discussions were cut short, some decisions postponed, others hastily made, and we all waited for a break in the rain and retired to our thatch houses. Everyone knew cement and zinc buildings were hot and noisy, but very few community centers and gathering places were still made with the traditional thatch and board, which people commonly described as cooler and quieter. Development monies from various sources were commonly provided to communities, albeit at random intervals, from various sources for projects such as building community centers. Zinc and cement houses were more expensive but generally considered to be an improvement, accompanied by a narrative of permanence and comfort. On that day and many others like it, my sensory experience illuminated how this sort of development—a movement away from the traditional practice of making a thatch house—had potentially undermined the practice of the *ab'ink*. Listening is incredibly important for reaching collective decisions, as is the maintenance of a calm demeanor. When people feel frustrated, hot, tired, and unable to hear, it is easy to see the potential to erode the process.

Similar to critiques of biomedicine, critiques of development are not difficult to find. However, like the biomedical model, the hegemonic global development model persists.[23] Increased pressures to attend high school, to grow commodity crops, to birth in the hospital, to use hybrid seeds, to buy rather than make food, to take pills and get injections, and more are associated with the assumption that moving along a linear pathway to "modernity"

---

23. At the time of writing, there are observable shifts in the global economic system and management of international resources away from a U.S./Eurocentric focus, in part in response to this hegemonic privileging of this ideological focus and exertion of force in service of it.

is a desired and inevitable consequence of living in a changing world. The "development assumption"—people need it, people want it, it is inherently connected to the pursuit of a better life—is pervasive, yet people develop counternarratives, valuing traditional knowledge and returning to the practices of home. These practices present a challenge to assimilation models of immigrant health in the United States and exploit the opportunities of the urban environment.[24] Communities keep spaces to support their cultural traditions and their well-being, picking and choosing from the "development" they are offered, and that which they seek.

COLLECTIVE HEALING AND HISTORICAL TRAUMA

When Rosita invited me to join her and a small group of Garifuna ladies at the St. Vincent heritage celebration in Brooklyn, and when she reminded me, "We experience good health when we come together to talk," she encapsulated one of the main findings of this research. As the ladies joined in and continued to explain how listening and sharing stories with each other keeps their culture alive and also keeps them well, I thought back to the last decade traveling back and forth to Belize. A few months earlier, I had a similar conversation in the very different setting of Santa Cruz. Sitting with the ladies in her extended family, Felicitas shared what she thought was the most important practice for maintaining health: "It's good to talk to each other." I have learned more than it is possible to articulate from these two women in their seventh decade of life—one Garifuna, one Q'eqchi' Maya—both of whom have built great lives through remarkable changes while carrying the adversities that their families and their ancestors had experienced with them. I

---

24. Ogilvie and Harrod discuss Alaskan Natives in urban environments, and how this benefits their health through the maintenance of traditions in this environment.

have always shared with my undergraduate students that social relationships were found to be the most critical factor to health and happiness.[25] Now, with the COVID-19 pandemic in between these discussions and my writing this, the importance of talking to each other has never been more palpable in the popular consciousness. The increased attention to mental health and the detrimental effects of loneliness and isolation are discussed across every forum. Humans are social: we all need someone to talk to. It is very difficult to stay healthy in isolation.[26]

"Our people have experienced trauma. We have all experienced trauma." I am sitting again with Pablo Miis, this time in his home in Punta Gorda, thinking through some of the lessons and challenges of the Maya communities' desire to interface with the wider Belizean and international communities, while still recognizing the value of their traditions. Pablo's comment resonated with my research exploring how epigenetics is mitigated by the sensory in relation to historical trauma. He applied academic language to a relationship Maya and Garifuna stories of health have illuminated quite clearly. The pressures to explain, justify, and maintain a way of life that prioritizes Indigenous values and practices is challenging in an increasingly changing world where global economic priorities are reflected in cultural practices. Colonial legacies are carried in bodies in a generational sense, but often these traumas are reinforced through daily reminders, both small and larger. Listening to the radio, something I have done with both Maya and Garifuna community members, often brings reminders of how traditional values have been, and continue to be, challenged. Stories of crime, social

---

25. *Time Magazine* has published many popular articles based on studies relating happiness to positive social relationships, notably on March 7, 2014 ("6 Secrets You Can Learn from the Happiest People on Earth"). Indigenous people have known and practiced these connections for generations. As an example, Stephenson (2014) addresses social relationships in Indigenous arctic communities in the context of care.

26. See Baines's 2020 op-ed, "Health Is More than the Absence of Disease: An Important Coronavirus Lesson" (in *Daily News*, April 22, 2020).

isolation and disconnection from the land, disputed land claims, language loss all contribute to reinforcing historical trauma. But sensory experiences make it better. Access to land to continue traditional farming and wild harvesting practices make it better. Supporting song and dance in community makes it better. There is strong agreement that heritage practices make it better.

These pathways are not always linear. Sometimes change for better at first reinforces and deepens historical trauma. During the testimony in support of Maya land rights, Maya people have consistently faced opposition to practices they have carried out for centuries. On the homecoming trip to Balliceaux, and in similar reminders across social media, Garifuna people have faced the stark realities of a centuries-old genocide, reliving those traumas of the ancestors as they struggled to survive. Collective memory, when performed and practiced, is both painful and healing. The collective energy of the sensory practice, through dance, through music, through working together, has efficacy in healing. "Get on the dance floor to heal inherited trauma."[27] Although my research—and indeed research since Durkheim and likely before—supports this collective response to trauma, the biomedical model continues to focus on the individual. But a full consideration of health and wellness shows that the focus on the individual—both in terms of patient and practitioner—is a large part of the problem.[28] Focusing on the individual as an exclusive solution is misguided. Collective experiences mitigated in individual bodies illuminate healing pathways.

---

27. Le Baron (2023) discussed the power of collective movement in relation to his work with inner city youth in East London at the Green Templeton College Conference for Human Welfare.

28. Watts (2023) discussed the need for elders in healing traditions and a movement away from this practice in what she critiques as our current "century of the self" at the Green Templeton College Conference for Human Welfare.

FOLLOWING THE PLANTS

I was headed south on the bus along the Hummingbird Highway when a uniformed Kriol man sat beside me. As he struck up a conversation, I learned that he worked in a government agency. He wondered where I was headed and what I was up to. As I explained a little about my research, he, unexpectedly, began to share his extensive knowledge of local plants and what they might be used for. A few minutes into our conversation, the bus stopped to let passengers off, and he pointed to several of the plants he had just mentioned along the roadside. He was excited to share his thoughts on the benefits of botanical medicines and the details of what each was traditionally used for. I scribbled in my notebook, keen to cross-reference my knowledge gained from the Maya and Garifuna communities and to learn some new plants as well. Before he disembarked, I learned that his daughter was abroad attending medical school, and I asked him if he had taught her about all these plant medicines he had shared with me. He shrugged and smiled, and I considered how often knowledge systems and practices so often set in opposition coexisted in my research encounters—and in the daily lives of people. Approaches to healthcare and well-being are pluralistic, with people choosing modalities that "make sense" and "resonate in visceral as well as cognitive ways."[29]

When I explain that this book, and my research in general, explores the intersections of health, ecology, and tradition through a sensory lens, people most commonly assume that my study centers around ethnobotanicals, or plant medicines. Traditional medicinal practices are employed in significant ways among both Maya and Garifuna communities. Many of these are documented in the preceding chapters; however, my aim is not to provide a comprehensive account of the extensive ethnobotanical knowledge held throughout Belize. Plants and

---

29. See Good (2018) for a discussion of the intersection of the sensory and the cognitive ways of understanding healthcare modalities and Resser's (2014) work on healthcare pluralism in southern Belize.

plant medicines are an important part of how the communities represented here interact with the natural world—and find their place within it. I came to understand this by following the stories of the plants as they intersected with the stories of the people documented here. Often the stories led me to a sensory experience: harvesting the plants—walking in the forest, noticing, feeling, pulling; processing the plants—boiling, smelling, hearing, seeing the water change color; administering the plants—drinking, tasting the bitterness, wrapping and rubbing, feeling coolness on the skin, the heat of the swelling. The relationships with the plants and their traditional preparations kept the people grounded in their natural bodies. The plants served as reminders of their mother's wisdom, their auntie's healing, and their grandma's longevity. The plants were more than their chemical properties—they were teachers, helpers, old friends, always there, even in times of change.

THE DANCE GOES ON

I walked through the security scanners and all the way around the building to reach the entrance to the main staircase. I stared up at the ornate lofted ceilings as I gave my name. Rosita had put me on the list for the event, the closing ceremony for Garifuna Heritage month in New York City, held in the council chambers at the city hall. As I climbed the stairs and entered the chambers, I was immediately struck by the swath of yellow that stood in contrast to the dark wood fixtures. The community had come out, many dressed in the colors of the Garifuna flag, yellow, white, and black, configured on cloth with vibrant patterns and tailoring ranging from high fashion to "traditional." Having yet to get my traditional clothes, I felt muted and underdressed. As the proceedings began, I listened to the narratives of entrepreneurship and celebrated the successes of the honorees, Garifuna New Yorkers representing their community with excellence. While I thought about (and silently critiqued) the standard of success at play in this space, out came the Jankunu dancers,

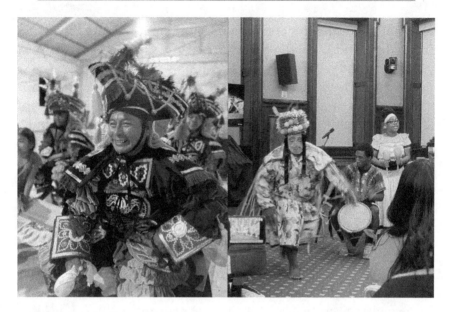

FIGURE 12 (left) Maya Deer Dancer, Basilio Teul, Santa Cruz, Toledo, Belize and (right) Garifuna Jankunu Dancer, New York City Hall. Kristina Baines.

mocking the colonizers with their colorful costumes and masks of white face.[30] I thought about how this dance, performed in 2023 inside the two-hundred-year-old halls of government in the largest city in the United States, had persisted with very little change over the centuries of Garifuna celebrations.

A few months later, back in Santa Cruz, I watched as Basilio donned the white-faced mask of the general in a performance of the Deer Dance. Like the Jankunu dancers, the Deer Dancers harnessed the joy in the mockery of the colonizers. This came through their sensory experiences: the percussive music— rhythmic and repetitive—with instruments crafted from materials from the forest, trees carved and polished. Rhythmic and

---

30. The Jankunu (also Junkanoo) is a dance with roots in enslaved African communities performed in several countries of the English-speaking Caribbean and US settlements of those West Indian communities, including Belize, Jamaica, and the Bahamas. It is considered a traditional dance for Garifuna communities, particularly in Belize.

repetitive like the dances, swaying, jumping, turning, back and forth, over and over, the colorful costumes and masks, not just pale faces but yellows and reds and patterns and mirrors, mesmerizing and reminding the spectators of their relationships with both the natural world and those who sought to disrupt that relationship through the extraction of resources, through displacement. I thought about both the subtle distinctions in the observations and arguments I have made during the years spent learning from Maya and Garifuna communities, and also the most reductive of tropes: the more things change, the more they stay the same.

THE CHANGING LANGUAGE OF HEALTH

I was visiting Santa Cruz for just a short time in 2018, but I had been enlisted to help bake tortillas for a wedding hosted by my longtime neighbors and friends. As I sat, once again, on a low stool, my hands gently and knowingly shaping the corn masa, a young child—maybe three years old—ran up to the table to speak to his mother, who was baking tortillas next to me. This was common in my many years of tortilla-making, and I was accustomed to seeing the small faces curiously looking at me. This time, however, I was struck, prompted to look up from my mesmerizing practice. The child had approached and addressed his mother in English. In the past, children would not typically learn English until they started school at age five or six. I inquired and was told that they spoke English at home, too. I was surprised, as language loss had not been identified as a critical issue among Maya communities in the same way it had with Garifuna communities I worked with. Perhaps that was changing.

I had been told many times by Maya and Garifuna people alike that the most important part of traditional practice to keep is the language. This was not a systematic ranking or assessment of the most important traditional practice, and oftentimes, the same people emphasized that working together was the most important traditional practice. Many times these went hand in hand. English words cutting across a sea of Mopan chatter, however, did seem like a very stark reminder of the ongoing colonial legacies noticeable in everyday practices.

As I hope I have made clear throughout this book, I did not set out to write an indictment of the forces of change thrust upon Indigenous communities as part of the global colonial project. These are well-documented.[31] This book does challenge the popular internalizing of the primacy of Western epistemologies that persist even amid the rhetoric of decolonization. This persistence is especially evident in discussions around global development and definitions of science. These ethnographic accounts speak to these discussions and definitions. The stories shared here are not about communities who desire to exclude technology or romanticize tradition. They are the stories of people who, through varied and ever-responsive ways, embody their traditional values and continue their traditional practices because they work in the context of building healthy, everyday lives. Health and healing are woven into every aspect of daily practice. There is change and there is loss, but there is persistence and there is joy and there is healing.

---

31. Simpson (2007) illustrates how "culture" within anthropology remains a categorization of difference as compared to the unquestioned core self of empire, thus serving as a key technology of governance and discipline of space, resources, and bodies. Critiques of both the colonial project at large, and anthropology's role in it, are plentiful. See Deloria Jr. (1988), Castro-Gomez (2008), and Coronil (2000) for relevant discussion.

REFERENCES

Abel, S., and C. J. Frieman. 2023. "On Gene-ealogy: Identity, Descent, and Affiliation in the Era of Home DNA Testing." *Anthropological Science* 131 (1): 15–25.

Appah, N. 2018. "Assessing the Impact of Coastal Resort Tourism on Tourism Participation Among the Locals in Hopkins Village, Belize." Master's thesis, University of Manitoba. Available at http://hdl.handle.net/1993/33605.

Baines, K. 2001. "The Nature of Nature: South Floridian Children and Their Environmental Experience." MA thesis, Florida Atlantic University.

Baines, K. 2016a. *Embodying Ecological Heritage in a Maya Community: Health, Happiness, and Identity.* Lanham, Md.: Lexington Books.

Baines, K. 2016b. "The Environmental Heritage and Wellness Assessment: Applying Quantitative Techniques to Traditional Ecological Knowledge and Wellness Relationships." *Journal of Ecological Anthropology* 18 (1).

Baines, K. 2018. "But Are They Actually Healthier?: Challenging the Health/Wellness Divide Through the Ethnography of Embodied Ecological Heritage." *Medicine Anthropology Theory* 5 (5): 5–29.

Baines, K. 2023. "Embodying the Everyday: Health and Heritage Practice Relationships in Latin American and Caribbean Immigrant Communities in New York City." *Human Organization* 82 (4): 331–41.

Baines, K. Forthcoming. "Decolonial Methodologies: Lessons from the Ab'ink."

Baines, K., and V. Costa, eds. 2022. *Cool Anthropology: How to Engage the Public with Academic Research.* Toronto: University of Toronto Press.

Baines, K., and P. Miis. 2024. "'It's Good for the Forest and It's Traditional': Indigenous Ecologies and Land Management at the Community/NGO

Interface in Southern Belize." *Culture, Agriculture, Food and Environment* 46 (1): 11–22.

Baines, K., and T. Rahman. Forthcoming. "Mapping Health and Happiness in a Maya Community."

Baines, K., and R. K. Zarger. 2012. "Circles of Value: Integrating Maya Environmental Knowledge into Belizean Schools." In *The Anthropology of Environmental Education*, edited by H. Kopnina, 25–46. Hauppauge, N.Y.: Nova Science Publishers.

Baines, K., and R. Zarger. 2017. "'It's Good to Learn About the Plants': Promoting Social Justice and Community Health Through the Development of a Maya Environmental and Cultural Heritage Curriculum in Southern Belize." *Journal of Environmental Studies and Sciences* 7 (3): 416–24.

Benson, M., and N. Osbaldiston, eds. 2014. *Understanding Lifestyle Migration: Theoretical Approaches to Migration and the Quest for a Better Way of Life*. Houndsmith, Basingstoke: Palgrave Macmillan.

Biglin, J. 2020. "Embodied and Sensory Experiences of Therapeutic Space: Refugee Place-Making Within an Urban Allotment." *Health & Place* 62:102309.

Black Elk, L. 2016. "Native Science: Understanding and Respecting Other Ways of Thinking." *Rangelands* 38 (1): 3–4.

Booher, A., and K. Oths, dirs. 2018. *The Last Bonesetter: An Encounter with Don Felipe*. Documentary Educational Resources.

Borgatti, S. P. 1996. *Anthropac 4.0*. Analytic Technologies.

Brettell, C. B. 2014. "Theorizing Migration in Anthropology: The Cultural, Social, and Phenomenological Dimensions of Movement." In *Migration Theory*, edited by C. B. Brettell and J. F. Hollifield, 148–97. London: Routledge.

Bruce-Keller, A.J., J. M. Salbaum, and H. R. Berthoud. 2018. "Harnessing Gut Microbes for Mental Health: Getting from Here to There." *Biological Psychiatry* 83 (3): 214–23.

Cantor, A. R., I. Chan, and K. Baines. 2018. "From the Chacra to the Tienda: Dietary Delocalization in the Peruvian Andes." *Food and Foodways* 26 (3): 198–222.

Capaldi, C. A., R. L. Dopko, and J. M. Zelenski. 2014. "The Relationship Between Nature Connectedness and Happiness: A Meta-Analysis." *Frontiers in Psychology* 5.

Castañeda, H. 2010. "Im/migration and Health: Conceptual, Methodological, and Theoretical Propositions for Applied Anthropology." *Napa Bulletin* 34 (1): 6–27.

Castañeda, H., 2020. *Borders of Belonging: Struggle and Solidarity in Mixed-Status Immigrant Families*. Stanford: Stanford University Press.

Castañeda, H., S. M. Holmes, D. S. Madrigal, M. E. D. Young, N. Beyeler, and J. Quesada. 2015. "Immigration as a Social Determinant of Health." *Annual Review of Public Health* 36:375–92.

Castro-Gomez, S. 2008. "(Post)Coloniality for Dummies: Latin American Perspectives on Modernity, Coloniality, and the Geopolitics of Knowledge." In *Coloniality at Large: Latin America and the Postcolonial Debate*, edited by M. Moraña, E. Dussel, and C. A. Jáuregui, 259–85. Durham, N.C.: Duke University Press.

Chan, S. C. 2005. "Temple-Building and Heritage in China." *Ethnology* 44 (1): 65–79.

Collins, R. 2014. "Interaction Ritual Chains and Collective Effervescence." In *Collective Emotions: Perspectives from Psychology, Philosophy, and Sociology*, edited by C. von Scheve and M. Salmela, 299–311. Oxford: Oxford University Press.

Coronil, F. 2000. "Towards a Critique of Globalcentrism: Speculations on Capitalism's Nature." *Public Culture* 12 (2): 251–374.

Cortez, C., L. Pacheco-Cobos, B. Culleton, M. Grote. 2017. *The Effect of Fallow, Soil Nutrients and Site Properties on Mayan Maize Yields in the Milpa Agroecosystem of Santa Cruz, Belize*. Report, University of California, Davis.

Crane, T. A. 2010. "Of Models and Meanings: Cultural Resilience in Social–Ecological Systems." *Ecology and Society* 15 (4).

Cunin, E., and O. Hoffman. 2013. "From Colonial Domination to the Making of the Nation: Ethno-Racial Categories in Censuses and Reports and Their Political Uses in Belize, 19th–20th Centuries." *Caribbean Studies* 41 (2): 31–60.

Deloria, V., Jr. 1988. "Reflections on the Black Hills Claim." *Wicazo Sa Review* 4 (1): 33–38.

Dentzau, M. W. 2019. "The Tensions Between Indigenous Knowledge and Western Science." *Cultural Studies of Science Education* 14:1031–36.

Descola, P. 2006. "Beyond Nature and Culture." In *Proceedings of the British Academy* 139:137–55.

Downey, G. 2002. "Listening to Capoeira: Phenomenology, Embodiment, and the Materiality of Music." *Ethnomusicology* 46 (3): 487–509.

Dressler, W., K. Oths, M. C. Balieiro, R. P. Ribeiro, and J. E. Dos Santos. 2012. "How Culture Shapes the Body: Cultural Consonance and Body Mass in Urban Brazil." *American Journal of Human Biology* 24 (3): 325–31.

Dressler, W. W., K. S. Oths, and C. C. Gravlee. 2005. "Race and Ethnicity in Public Health Research: Models to Explain Health Disparities." *Annual Review of Anthropology* 34:231–52.

England, S. 2023. *Afro Central Americans in New York City: Garifuna Tales of Transnational Movements in Racialized Space*. Gainesville: University Press of Florida.

Enriquez, J., ed. 2017. *To Educate a Nation: Autobiography of Andres P. and Jane V. Enriquez*. Caye Caulker, Belize: Producciones de La Hamaca.

Escobar, A. 1995. *Encountering Development: The Making and Unmaking of the Third World*. Princeton, N.J.: Princeton University Press.

Fassin, D. 2007. *When Bodies Remember: Experiences and Politics of AIDS in South Africa*. Berkeley: University of California Press.

Finerman, R., and R. Sackett. 2003. "Using Home Gardens to Decipher Health and Healing in the Andes." *Medical Anthropology Quarterly* 17 (4): 459–82.

Finneran, N., and C. Welch. 2020. "Mourning Balliceaux: Towards a Biography of a Caribbean Island of Death, Grief and Memory." *Island Studies Journal* 15 (2): 1–18.

Fischer, E. F. 2014. *The Good Life: Aspiration, Dignity, and the Anthropology of Wellbeing*. Stanford: Stanford University Press.

Foster, G. M. 1979. "Humoral Traces in United States Folk Medicine." *Medical Anthropology Newsletter* 10 (2): 17–20.

Fuller, K. S., and C. Torres Rivera. 2021. "A Culturally Responsive Curricular Revision to Improve Engagement and Learning in an Undergraduate Microbiology Lab Course." *Frontiers in Microbiology* 11:577852.

Fuller, S., and J. H. Collier. 2003. *Philosophy, Rhetoric, and the End of Knowledge: A New Beginning for Science and Technology Studies*. London: Routledge.

Fuster, M., and E. González. 2019. "Traditional Diets in Everyday Life: Perspectives from Hispanic Caribbean Communities in New York City." *Food and Foodways* 27 (4): 316–37.

Galla, C., and A. Holmes. 2020. "Indigenous Thinkers: Decolonizing and Transforming the Academy Through Indigenous Relationality." In *Decolonizing and Indigenizing Education in Canada*, edited by S. Cote-Meek and T. Moeke-Pickering, 51–71. Toronto: Canadian Scholars.

Gálvez, A. 2018. *Eating NAFTA: Trade, Food Policies, and the Destruction of Mexico*. Oakland: University of California Press.

Gálvez, A. 2019. "Transnational Mother Blame: Protecting and Caring in a Globalized Context." *Medical Anthropology* 38 (7): 574–87.

Garth, H. 2023. "Food, Taste, and the Body: Ingestion and Embodiment in Santiago de Cuba." *Medical Anthropology Quarterly* 37 (1): 5–22.

Gebara, M. F. 2023. "What Is Medicine? Indigenous Rituals, Amazonian Ontologies, and the Psychedelic Renaissance." Paper presented at Green Templeton College, Conference for Human Welfare, Oxford, May 15, 2023.

Gómez-Barris, M. 2017. *The Extractive Zone: Social Ecologies and Decolonial Perspectives*. Durham, N.C.: Duke University Press.

Gone, J. P. 2013. "Redressing First Nations Historical Trauma: Theorizing Mechanisms for Indigenous Culture as Mental Health Treatment." *Transcultural Psychiatry* 50 (5): 683–706.

González, V. M., and L. A. Castro. 2007. "Keeping Strong Connections to the Homeland via Web-Based Tools: The Case of Mexican Migrant Communities in the United States." *Journal of Community Informatics* 3 (3): 1–27.

Good, B. 2018. "Making Sense and Sensation." In *Capturing Quicksilver: The Position, Power, and Plasticity of Chinese Medicine in Singapore*, edited by A. A. Smith, 144–78. New York: Berghahn.

Gow, D. D. 2002. "Anthropology and Development: Evil Twin or Moral Narrative?" *Human Organization* 61 (4): 299–313.

Greene, N. 1972. *Hegel on the Soul: A Speculative Anthropology*. The Hauge: Nijhoff.

Haila, Y. 2000. "Beyond the Nature-Culture Dualism." *Biology and Philosophy* 15:155–75.

Haines, S. 2018. "Imagining the Highway: Anticipating Infrastructural and Environmental Change in Belize." *Ethnos* 83 (2): 392–413.

Hall, E., and N. G. Cuellar. 2016. "Immigrant Health in the United States: A Trajectory Toward Change." *Journal of Transcultural Nursing* 27 (6): 611–26.

Halliburton, M. 2002. "Rethinking Anthropological Studies of the Body: Manas and Bōdham in Kerala." *American Anthropologist* 104 (4): 1123–34.

Hatala, A. R., and J. B. Waldram. 2015. "The Role of Sensorial Processes in Q'eqchi' Maya Healing: A Case Study of Depression and Bereavement." *Transcultural Psychiatry* 53 (1): 60–80.

Hatala, A. R., and J. B. Waldram. 2017. "Diagnostic Emplotment in Q'eqchi' Maya Medicine." *Medical Anthropology* 36 (3): 273–86.

Hernandez, A., A. K. Hurtig, M. San Sebastian, F. Jerez, and W. Flores. 2022. "'History Obligates Us to Do It': Political Capabilities of Indigenous Grassroots Leaders of Health Accountability Initiatives in Rural Guatemala." *BMJ Global Health* 7 (5): 1–12.

Hsu, E. 2007. "The Biocultural in the Cultural: The Five Agents and the Body Ecologic in Chinese Medicine." In *Holistic Anthropology: Emergence and Convergence*, edited by D. Parkin and S. J. Ulijaszek, 91–126. New York: Berghahn Books.

Hsu, E. 2017. "Durkheim's Effervescence and Its Maussian Afterlife in Medical Anthropology." *Durkheimian Studies* 23 (1): 76–105.

Hsu, E., 2022. *Chinese Medicine in East Africa: An Intimacy with Strangers*. New York: Berghahn Books.

Ingold, T., 2020. *Correspondences*. Hoboken, N.J.: John Wiley & Sons.

Ingold, T. 2021. *The Perception of the Environment: Essays on Livelihood, Dwelling and Skill*. London: Routledge.

Izquierdo, C. 2005. "When 'Health' Is Not Enough: Societal, Individual and Biomedical Assessments of Well-Being Among the Matsigenka of the Peruvian Amazon." *Social Science & Medicine* 61 (4): 767–83.

Järbrink-Sehgal, E., and A. Andreasson. 2020. "The Gut Microbiota and Mental Health in Adults." *Current Opinion in Neurobiology* 62:102–14.

Johnson, M. A. 2019. *Becoming Creole: Nature and Race in Belize.* New Brunswick, N.J.: Rutgers University Press.

Joseph, M. 2020. "Islands, History, and Decolonial Memory." *Island Studies Journal* 15 (2): 193–200.

Katz, R. 1982. *Boiling Energy: Community Healing Among the Kalahari Kung.* Cambridge, Mass.: Harvard University Press.

Katz, R. 1984. "Empowerment and Synergy: Expanding the Community's Healing Resources." In *Studies in Empowerment: Steps toward Understanding and Action*, edited by J. Rappaport, C. Swift, and R. Hess, 201–26. New York: Haworth Press.

Kim, J. 2010. "Neighborhood Disadvantage and Mental Health: The Role of Neighborhood Disorder and Social Relationships." *Social Science Research* 39 (2): 260–71.

Kimmerer, R. 2020. *Braiding Sweetgrass: Indigenous Wisdom, Scientific Knowledge and the Teachings of Plants.* Minneapolis: Milkweed Editions.

Kirksey, S. E., and S. Helmreich. 2010. "The Emergence of Multispecies Ethnography." *Cultural Anthropology* 25 (4): 545–76.

Komito, L. 2011. "Social Media and Migration: Virtual Community 2.0." *Journal of the American Society for Information Science and Technology* 62 (6): 1075–86.

Ko'omoa, D. L. T., and A. K. Maunakea. 2017. "Linking Hawaiian Concepts of Health with Epigenetic Research: Implications in Developing Indigenous Scientists." In *Ho 'i Hou Ka Mauli Ola: Pathways to Native Hawaiian Health*, edited by W. K. Mesiona Lee and M. A. Look, 120–35. Honolulu: University of Hawai'i Press.

Koster, M. 2020. "An Ethnographic Perspective on Urban Planning in Brazil: Temporality, Diversity and Critical Urban Theory." *International Journal of Urban and Regional Research* 44 (2): 185–99.

Laderman, C., and M. Roseman, eds. 2016. *The Performance of Healing.* New York: Routledge.

Latour, B. 2017. "Anthropology at the Time of the Anthropocene: A Personal View of What Is to Be Studied." In *The Anthropology of Sustainability: Beyond Development and Progress*, edited by A. L. Tsing, M. Brigthman, and J. Lewis, 35–49. New York: Palgrave Macmillan.

Leatherman, T., and A. Goodman. 2005. "Coca-Colonization of Diets in the Yucatan." *Social Science & Medicine* 61 (4): 833–46.

Leatherman, T., and A. Goodman. 2020. "Building on the Biocultural Syntheses: 20 Years and Still Expanding." *American Journal of Human Biology* 32 (4): e23360.

Le Baron, D. 2023. "Diversity in Psychedelics." Paper presented at Green Templeton College Conference for Human Welfare, Oxford, May 15, 2023.

Lende, D. H. 2012. "Poverty Poisons the Brain." *Annals of Anthropological Practice* 36 (1): 183–201.

Levitt, P. 2010. "Transnationalism." In *Diasporas: Concepts, Intersections, Identities*, edited by J. Lesser et al., 39–44. London: Bloomsbury.

Lewis, S. L., and M. A. Maslin. 2015. "Defining the Anthropocene." *Nature* 519 (7542): 171–80.

Lock, M. 2015. "Comprehending the Body in the Era of the Epigenome." *Current Anthropology* 56 (2): 151–77.

Logan, M. 1975. "Selected References on the Hot-Cold Theory of Disease." *Medical Anthropology Newsletter* 6 (2): 8–14.

Mancinelli, F. 2021. "Lifestyle Migrations in the Asia Pacific: A Socio-Anthropological Review." Migration and Mobility in the Asia Pacific Working Paper no. 4, Monash University, Malaysia.

Marks, J. 2013. "The Nature/Culture of Genetic Facts." *Annual Review of Anthropology* 42:247–67.

Marx, K. 1992 [1844]. "Economic and Philosophical Manuscripts." In *Early Writings*, translated by R. Livingstone and G. Benton, 279–400. New York: Penguin Classics.

McDade, T. W. 2002. "Status Incongruity in Samoan Youth: A Biocultural Analysis of Culture Change, Stress, and Immune Function." *Medical Anthropology Quarterly* 16 (2): 123–50.

Medina, L. K. 2003. "Commoditizing Culture: Tourism and Maya Identity." *Annals of Tourism Research* 30 (2): 353–68.

Messer, E. 1987. "The Hot and Cold in Mesoamerican Indigenous and Hispanicized Thought." *Social Science & Medicine* 25:339–46.

Moerman, D. 2002. *Meaning, Medicine, and the "Placebo Effect."* Cambridge: Cambridge University Press.

Moore, A. 2016. "Anthropocene Anthropology: Reconceptualizing Contemporary Global Change." *Journal of the Royal Anthropological Institute* 22 (1): 27–46.

Moran-Thomas, A. 2019. *Traveling with Sugar: Chronicles of a Global Epidemic*. Oakland: University of California Press.

Mosse, D. 2013. "The Anthropology of International Development." *Annual Review of Anthropology* 42:227–46.

Mundel, E., and G. E. Chapman. 2010. "A Decolonizing Approach to Health Promotion in Canada: The Case of the Urban Aboriginal Community Kitchen Garden Project." *Health Promotion International* 25 (2): 166–73.

Narby, J. 2005. *Intelligence in Nature: An Inquiry into Knowledge*. New York: Penguin.

Neveling, P. 2017. "The Political Economy Machinery: Toward a Critical Anthropology of Development as a Contested Capitalist Practice." *Dialectical Anthropology* 41 (2): 163–83.

Nichter, M. 2008. "Coming to Our Senses: Appreciating the Sensorial in Medical Anthropology." *Transcultural Psychiatry* 45 (2): 163–97.

Noble, D. 2013. "Physiology Is Rocking the Foundations of Evolutionary Biology." *Experimental Physiology* 98 (8): 1235–43.
Noble, D. 2017. *Dance to the Tune of Life: Biological Relativity*. Cambridge: Cambridge University Press.
Noble, D. 2022. "Modern Physiology Vindicates Darwin's Dream." *Experimental Physiology* 107 (9): 1015–28.
Nolan, R. W. 2018. *Development Anthropology: Encounters in the Real World*. Boulder: Westview Press.
Noone, M. J. 2020. "Music and the 'World of Feeling.'" In *Phenomenologies of Grace: The Body, Embodiment, and Transformative Futures*, 257–71, edited by M. Bussey and C. Mozzini-Alister. London: Palgrave Macmillan.
O'Donnell, J., D. Cárdenas, N. Orazani, A. Evans, and K. J. Reynolds. 2022. "The Longitudinal Effect of COVID-19 Infections and Lockdown on Mental Health and the Protective Effect of Neighbourhood Social Relations." *Social Science & Medicine* 297:114821.
Oro, P. J. L. 2020. "Garifunizando Ambas Américas: Hemispheric Entanglements of Blackness/Indigeneity/AfroLatinidad." *Postmodern Culture* 31 (1).
Palacio, Joseph O., Judy Lumb, and Carlson Tuttle. 2009. "Transmission of Rights to House Lots in Barranco, a Garifuna Village in Southern Belize 1895 to 2000.—Lessons in Caribbean Ethnohistory." In *Ethnicidad y nación: Debate alrededor de Belice / Belize: Ethnicity and Nation*, coord. Elisabeth Cunin and Odile Hoffman, 87–115.
Palacio, M. 2023. "Belize @42—Time for the Redefinition of Ethnicity." Presented at the Belize KULCHA Symposium, September 8, 2023.
Paranich, M. 2018. "Anthropological Futures for the Study of Cultural Resilience of 'Western' Societies in the Face of Climate Change." *COMPASS* 2 (1): 18–35.
Peller, H. A. 2021. "Soil Fertility, Agroecology, and Social Change in Southern Belize." PhD diss., Ohio State University.
Pelto, G. H., and P. J. Pelto. 1983. "Diet and Delocalization: Dietary Changes Since 1750." *Journal of Interdisciplinary History* 14 (2): 507–28.
Piot, C. 1999. *Remotely Global: Village Modernity in West Africa*. Chicago: University of Chicago Press.
Prufer, K. M., A. E. Thompson, and D. J. Kennett. 2015. "Evaluating Airborne LiDAR for Detecting Settlements and Modified Landscapes in Disturbed Tropical Environments at Uxbenká, Belize." *Journal of Archaeological Science* 57:1–13.
Pugh, J. 2014. "Resilience, Complexity and Post-Liberalism." *Area* 46 (3): 313–19.
Pugh, J., 2021. "Resilience." In *Words and Worlds: A Lexicon for Dark Times*, edited by V. Dass and D. Fassin, chap. 11. Durham, N.C.: Duke University Press.

Rappaport, R. A. 1971. "Ritual, Sanctity, and Cybernetics." *American Anthropologist* 73 (1): 59–76.
Redvers, N. D. 2019. *The Science of the Sacred: Bridging Global Indigenous Medicine Systems and Modern Scientific Principles.* Berkeley, CA: North Atlantic Books.
Reese, A. M. 2018. "Food Access in the United States." In *Gender: Space*, Macmillan Interdisciplinary Handbooks, Gender Series, edited by A. M. Cox, 199–208. Farmington Hills, Mich.: Macmillan Reference.
Reeser, D. C. 2014. "Medical Pluralism in a Neoliberal State: Health and Deservingness in Southern Belize." PhD diss., University of South Florida.
Reyes-García, V., V. Vadez, S. Tanner, T. McDade, T. Huanca, and W. Leonard. 2006. "Evaluating Indices of Traditional Ecological Knowledge: A Methodological Contribution." *Journal of Ethnobiology and Ethnomedicine* 2: no pagination.
Rimé, B., and D. Páez. 2023. "Why We Gather: A New Look, Empirically Documented, at Émile Durkheim's Theory of Collective Assemblies and Collective Effervescence." *Perspectives on Psychological Science* 18 (6): 1306–30.
Schmidt, M. 2022. "Cultivating Health: Diabetes Resilience Through Neo-Traditional Farming in Mopan Maya Communities of Belize." *Agriculture and Human Values* 39 (1): 269–79.
Schuller, M. 2009. "Gluing Globalization: NGOs as Intermediaries in Haiti." *PoLAR: Political and Legal Anthropology Review* 32 (1): 84–104.
Shelton, B. L., and J. Marks. 2001. "Genetic Markers Not a Valid Test of Native Identity." Indigenous Peoples Council on Biocolonialism, http://www.ipcb.org/publications/briefing_papers/files/identity.html.
Shepherd, R. 2002. "Commodification, Culture and Tourism." *Tourist Studies* 2 (2): 183–201.
Simpson, A. 2007. "On Ethnographic Refusal: Indigeneity, 'Voice' and Colonial Citizenship." *Junctures: The Journal for Thematic Dialogue* 9:67–80.
Singer, M., and H. Baer. 2018. *Critical Medical Anthropology*. 2nd edition. New York: Routledge.
Sjöstedt-Hughes, P. 2023. "On the Need for Metaphysics in Psychedelic Therapy and Research." Paper presented at Green Templeton College Conference for Human Welfare, Oxford, May 15, 2023.
Smith, L. T. 1999. *Decolonizing Methodologies: Research and Indigenous Peoples*. London: Zed Books.
Spang, L. H. 2019. *Bite yu finga!: Innovating Belizean Cuisine*. Kingston, Jamaica: University of West Indies Press.
Staiano, K. V. 2016. *Interpreting Signs of Illness: A Case Study in Medical Semiotics*. Berlin: Mouton de Gruyter.
Stanley, E. 2019. "Religious Conversion and the Decline of Environmental Ritual Narratives." *Journal for the Study of Religion, Nature & Culture* 13 (3): 266–85.

Stephenson, L. 2014. *Life Beside Itself: Imagining Care in the Canadian Arctic.* Oakland: University of California Press.

Ströbele-Gregor, J. 1996. "Culture and Political Practice of the Aymara and Quechua in Bolivia: Autonomous Forms of Modernity in the Andes." *Latin American Perspectives* 23 (2): 72–90.

Sutton, D. E. 2010. "Food and the Senses." *Annual Review of Anthropology* 39:209–23.

Tedlock, B. 1987. "An Interpretive Solution to the Problem of Humoral Medicine in Latin America." *Social Science & Medicine* 24 (12): 1069–83.

Thayer, Z. M., and A. L. Non. 2015. "Anthropology Meets Epigenetics: Current and Future Directions." *American Anthropologist* 117 (4): 722–35.

Thomas, D. A. 2019. *Political Life in the Wake of the Plantation: Sovereignty, Witnessing, Repair.* Durham, N.C.: Duke University Press.

Thompson, J. J., C. Ritenbaugh, M. and Nichter. 2009. "Reconsidering the Placebo Response from a Broad Anthropological Perspective." *Culture, Medicine, and Psychiatry* 33:112–52.

Todd, Z. 2015. "Indigenizing the Anthropocene." In *Art in the Anthropocene: Encounters Among Aesthetics, Politics, Environments and Epistemologies,* edited by H. Davis and E. Turpin, 241–54. https://library.oapen.org/handle/20.500.12657/33191.

Toledo Alcaldes Association. N.d. *The Future We Dream.* Punta Gorda, Belize: Toledo Alcaldes Association.

Tongco, M. D. C. 2007. "Purposive Sampling as a Tool for Informant Selection." *Ethnobotany Research & Applications* 5:147–58.

Tsing, A. L. 2013. "More than Human Sociality." *Anthropology and Nature* 14 (1): 27–42.

Tsosie, R. 2007. "Indigenous People and Environmental Justice: The Impact of Climate Change." *University of Colorado Law Review* 78:1625.

Tung, J., and Y. Gilad. 2013. "Social Environmental Effects on Gene Regulation." *Cellular and Molecular Life Sciences* 70 (22): 4323–39.

Turner, V. W. 1969. *The Ritual Process.* London: Routledge.

Tynan, L. 2021. "What Is Relationality? Indigenous Knowledges, Practices and Responsibilities with Kin." *Cultural Geographies* 28 (4): 597–610.

Van Gennep, A. 1909. *Les rites de passage.* Paris: Émile Nourry.

Viruell-Fuentes, E. A., P. Y. Miranda, and S. Abdulrahim, 2012. "More than Culture: Structural Racism, Intersectionality Theory, and Immigrant Health." *Social Science & Medicine* 75 (12): 2099–106.

Wainwright, J., S. Jiang, K. Mercer, and D. Liu. 2015. "The Political Ecology of a Highway Through Belize's Forested Borderlands." *Environment and Planning A: Economy and Space* 47 (4): 833–49.

Walshe-Roussel, B. 2014. "An Ethnobiological Investigation of Q'eqchi'Maya and Cree of Eeyou Istchee Immunomodulatory Therapies." PhD diss., Université d'Ottawa/University of Ottawa.

Warin, M., E. Kowal, and M. Meloni. 2020. "Indigenous Knowledge in a Postgenomic Landscape: The Politics of Epigenetic Hope and Reparation in Australia." *Science, Technology, & Human Values* 45 (1): 87–111.

Watts, R. 2023. "Community Nature-Based Psychedelic Integration Models." Green Templeton College Conference for Human Welfare, Oxford, May 15, 2023.

West, P., J. Igoe, and D. Brockington. 2006. "Parks and Peoples: The Social Impact of Protected Areas." *Annual Review of Anthropology* 35:251–77.

Wiedman, D. 2012. "Native American Embodiment of the Chronicities of Modernity: Reservation Food, Diabetes, and the Metabolic Syndrome Among the Kiowa, Comanche, and Apache." *Medical Anthropology Quarterly* 26 (4): 595–612.

Wilk, R. 1999. "'Real Belizean Food': Building Local Identity in the Transnational Caribbean." *American Anthropologist* 101 (2): 244–55.

Wilk, R., 2002. "Consumption, Human Needs, and Global Environmental Change." *Global Environmental Change* 12 (1): 5–13.

Wilk, R. ed., 2006. *Fast Food/Slow Food: The Cultural Economy of the Global Food System*. Lanham, MD: Rowman Altamira.

Wilson, A. C. 2005. "Reclaiming Our Humanity: Decolonization and the Recovery of Indigenous Knowledge." In *War and Border Crossings: Ethics When Cultures Clash*, edited by P. A. French and J. A. Short, 255–63. Lanham, Md.: Rowman & Littlefield.

Wilson, S. 2008. *Research Is Ceremony: Indigenous Research Methods*. Winnipeg: Fernwood.

Winter, K., and W. McClatchey, W. 2009. "The Quantum Co-evolution Unit: An Example of Awa (Kava—Piper methysticum G. Foster) in Hawaiian Culture." *Economic Botany* 63 (4): 353–62.

Wood, B., O. Williams, P. Baker, and G. Sacks. 2023. "Behind the 'Creative Destruction' of Human Diets: An Analysis of the Structure and Market Dynamics of the Ultra-Processed Food Manufacturing Industry and Implications for Public Health." *Journal of Agrarian Change* 23 (4): 811–43.

Zarger, R. K. 2009. "Mosaics of Maya Livelihoods: Readjusting to Global and Local Food Crises." *Napa Bulletin* 32 (1): 130–51.

Zarger, R. K. 2010. "Learning the Environment." In *The Anthropology of Learning in Childhood*, edited by D. F. Lancy, J. Bock, and S. Gaskins, 341–70. Walnut Creek, Calif.: AltaMira Press.

Zarger, R., and K. Baines. Forthcoming. "Everything and Nothing Has Changed: Maya Farming and Climate Change in Southern Belize."

Zharkevich, I. 2019. *Maoist People's War and the Revolution of Everyday Life in Nepal*. Cambridge: Cambridge University Press.

INDEX

anthropology, 6, 8, 15n17, 16–17, 125nn11–12, 137n126

Belize, 3, 39, 50, 56, 65, 67, 80, 85, 109, 130, 133; and agriculture, 31; and Belize City, 27, 33, 52; and Belize National Indigenous Council (BENIC), 21; and biomedical system, 24, 121; and Brooklyn, 53; and "bush medicine", 81; and Caye Caulker, 33; and Chinese communities, 54–55; and coastal communities, 35, 51, 54; and communities, 5–6, 21, 84, 122n8, 131; and cottage industries, 104n7; and COVID-19, 46, 108; and Creole, 51n1, 60, 64; and culture, 66; and diabetes, 18n22; and diaspora, 98, 112; and disease, 18; and environmental NGOs, 9; and ethnic groups, 23, 29n1, 61; and farming, 74; and food, 12n12, 35, 44, 62, 72; and freedom, 58; and government, 95, 119; and healers, 121; and health, 19, 57, 125; and identity, 52; and Indigenous peoples, 14, 21, 38, 40, 120, 125; and irrigation, 31; and land rights, 37–39; and localism, 8n5; and Los Angeles, 102–4, 110; and marginalization, 58; and Maya communities, 9, 11–12, 13n13, 14, 20, 22, 22n28, 32, 36, 45, 61, 64, 75, 77–78, 81, 95, 106, 115n2, 116, 128; and medicinal plants, 23, 93; and migration, 16, 19; and music, 66; and New York City, 5, 94, 110; and pan-Belizean identity, 104; and plants, 53; and politics, 92; and professionals, 23; and Santa Cruz, 31; southern, 7, 11, 14, 28, 36, 46, 75n4, 79, 82n15, 96, 104; and Stan Creek, 103; and Toledo, 105; and tourism, 92; and United States, 5–6, 10

Belize National Indigenous Council (BENIC), 21, 38

caldo, 28, 34, 41, 43, 69–73, 84, 91, 104, 124, 126

Caribbean, 12n12, 54, 63, 65, 95, 121, 135; and Afro-Caribbean communities, 57, 97; genocide, 51

Caribbean High Court of Justice, 31n2, 37n6, 38
Caribbean Sea, 4, 49, 97, 103, 116
cassava, 62, 65, 67, 70, 91, 96, 101–2, 106–7, 110n10, 111, 113
children, 3, 29, 35, 46–47, 52, 72, 84, 86–87, 90, 99–100, 102–3, 107, 109, 116, 136; and dance, 110; and families, 36; Mopan Maya, 6; and schooling, 7, 28, 30, 32, 110, 126; and storytelling, 66; young, 41
collective, 64, 68, 80, 98, 106; care, 109; decision-making, 79, 128–29; effervescence, 99n4; experience, 102; heritage, 101; identity, 43; labor, 39; land use, 21; Maya community, 34; memory, 99, 101, 112n12, 132; practice, 117; and property rights, 37n6; trauma, 117; rights, 37n6
colonization, 90, 112, 131, 137; coca, 11n10; and genocide, 51, 95; and government, 51; history, 23, 128; and knowledge, 128n22; logics, 38; systems, 45, 92
corn, 35, 44, 47, 73, 84, 113; dried, 75; farming of, 11, 31, 36, 64, 74, 76–80, 82, 118; game, 84; genetically modified, 12; hybrid, 75; masa, 136; and matambre, 74; and *poch* (corn masa), 47, 70; preparation of, 9; tortillas, 20, 28, 43, 62, 85n17
critical medical anthropology, 15n17, 127
cultural anthropology, 58
cultural commodification, 89
cultural domination, 8n4
cultural genocide, 12
cultural groups, 52
cultural heritage, 97, 119, 130
cultural expectations, 11n10

cultural festivals, 25
cultural identity, 17, 25n30, 58, 60, 112
cultural practices, 6, 53, 60, 95, 99, 110, 119, 131
cultural representation, 66
cultural resilience, 13n13
culture, 8, 77n8, 92, 95, 124–26

dance, 18, 62–63, 66, 85, 87, 92, 96, 98, 132, 134–36
Deer Dance, 85–88, 92
development, 8, 9n7, 12, 17, 26, 31, 45, 73, 75, 129; assumption, 130; bias, 35; critique, 36n5; and ecological heritage (EEH), 14n16, 15; and ethnic identity, 23n29; goals, 40; and globalization, 11, 137; and ideology, 8–10, 117; and progress, 29; projects, 13n13, 106, 128; resort, 33; resources, 56; tourist, 22, 22n27; values, 36

embodied ecological heritage (EEH), 13–15, 126
ecological connections, 122
ecological practices, 14–17, 19, 42, 64, 73, 106
ecological systems, 5, 7, 79–80, 117
ecology, 8, 18, 133
economic change, 5, 14, 16, 20–21
economic development, 6, 8n4, 9, 38, 38
economic disparity, 109–10, 111n11
economic factors, 20
economic forces, 15n17
economic marginalization, 22
economic opportunities, 10, 56, 96
economic practices, 20, 131
economic security, 11
economic sense, 79
economic systems, 92, 129n23

INDEX 153

environmental activist, 78
environmental change, 5, 13n15, 14, 16, 21, 74
environmental factors, 20, 120
environmental health, 5n1
environmental knowledge, 17, 21, 26, 28, 120
environmental practices, 20–21
environmental projects, 9
environmental resources, 22, 120

family, 8, 20, 33–34, 38, 44, 46, 67, 91; and adversity, 130–31; and Belize, 23, 28–29, 104; and cassava, 111; and change, 10, 56; and community, 23, 97, 107; and coastal towns, 10; and cultural practices, 6; dynamics, 17, 24, 43, 54, 65, 130; and employment, 36; and enterprises, 119; and farming, 31, 35, 65; and food, 9, 45, 47, 58, 80, 102; and health, 40; and historical trauma, 130–31; and livelihood practices, 16, 36, 92; and Maya peoples, 51, 70; and rituals, 104; and rural villages, 28; and Santa Cruz, 86–87; and social media, 108n8; and wellness, 76
farming, 46; and community, 31, 74, 75n4; poultry, 91; practices, 9, 14, 45, 73, 75, 77–78; small scale, 23; subsistence, 37, 45; systems, 74; traditional, 20–21, 132; ventures, 65; and wage labor, 36
fast-food chains, 12
food, 14, 16, 20, 66, 70, 80, 100–101, 118, 130; Belizean, 12n12, 29; costs of, 20; and disease, 113; and farming, 45; Garifuna, 63; "ground", 22, 91, 110; groups, 41, 102; and health, 40, 111n10; and industrial food systems, 78, 102; Maya, 29, 35, 62; and mental food, 102; and nutritional value, 34; and preferences, 60; and taste, 35n4; vegan, 112
food security, 11–12

Garifuna, 6–7, 22–23, 29n1, 50, 98; and Britain, 95, 112n12; and Catholicism, 61; and celebrations, 135; and cerasee (*Yamor*), 41n9, 93; and collectivity, 64; communities, 4–5, 10, 21–22, 26, 51, 54, 87, 100, 102, 104, 108, 120, 135–36; and cooking, 62, 110–12; culture of, 23, 96–97, 99–104, 108–10, 114; and Dangriga, 56; and diabetes, 54n4, 124; and diaspora, 63, 95, 98; and Doctor Arzu, 121; and fishing, 11, 102; and generations, 107; and genocide, 132; and health conceptions, 23–24, 99, 112–13, 125, 127, 131; heritage, 65–66, 103, 105, 108, 111, 114, 130, 134; history, 4, 22, 99, 105, 112; and Hopkins, 50; and hospitality, 103; and *hudut*, 58, 60, 71, 126; and identity, 52–53, 60; and knowledge, 103; and language, 63, 66n14, 96, 136; and Los Angeles, 95, 97–98, 110–11, 115; and medicine, 133; and music, 62, 66, 96, 99; and New York City, 52, 94, 98, 125, 134; and plants, 133; Settlement Day, 50; and traditions, 14, 57, 64–66, 96, 102–3, 107, 116; and values, 100, 106, 109; and *xan*, 44; and young people, 63, 99
global capitalism, 9n8, 120
global climate crisis, 77
global colonialism, 137

global development, 12, 117, 129, 137
global economic system, 129n23, 131
global environment, 5
global food crisis (2006–8), 13n13
global narrative, 29
global pandemic, 5
global politics, 17

happiness, 40–43
healing, 134, 137; and collective memory, 132; journey, 90; modalities, 125; and pathways, 132; and plant medicines, 82; practice, 23, 82n15, 84, 121, 126–27; process, 82n16; and sensory experience, 82; sessions, 24; traditional, 83, 117, 132n28
health, 8, 13, 26, 38, 61, 69, 76, 83, 95, 106, 116–17; behaviors, 15n17; benefits, 70; and caldo, 72; and clinic, 83; community, 9n8, 11, 24, 77, 115; definition of, 5n1, 17; and diet, 22, 112, 124; and ecological context, 7, 133; and environment, 24; experiences of, 5, 14, 33, 130; and food, 62, 111; and happiness, 40–41, 43; and healthcare access, 18; and healthcare practitioners, 18; and heritage, 15, 21, 35, 59; holistic, 122n8; and identity, 43n13, 56; immigrant, 57, 130; impact on, 15; and Indigenous communities, 113, 120; individual, 11; inequity, 119n3; interventions, 83; and land practices, 40; maintenance of, 14, 16–18, 34, 52–54, 60, 62–63, 70, 80, 83–84, 92, 99, 102, 109, 112, 122, 124–25, 127–28, 130, 137; and Maya communities, 14, 23, 42–43, 79, 81; mental, 41n11, 103, 112; and migrants, 19; and migration, 16; and nutrients, 71; outcomes, 18–19, 55, 84, 113,
120; professionals, 126; and promotion, 23; social, 5n1, 102; and social relationships, 131; systems, 127; and traditional practices, 16; and wellness practices, 23, 64, 132
heritage, 3, 78, 130; blended, 97; collective, 101; conceptualizing, 25; connections, 22n28; culinary, 62; cultural, 97; ecological, 14–15, 120, 126; fluidity of, 63; Garifuna, 65–66, 100, 103, 105, 111, 134; health, 21, 35, 42–43, 59; identity, 15, 62, 101, 119; Maya, 33, 40, 119; traditions, 21, 96
heritage practices, 17, 25, 28, 58, 61, 65, 73, 103, 106–8, 113, 115n2, 132; and commodification, 109; and consistency, 67, 109; and ecological systems, 5; and farming, 18; and food, 18, 107; and health, 15, 18; and identity, 11; Indigenous, 120; intensification of, 25; and Maya community members, 14, 33; and time, 55
high schools, 7, 28–29, 32, 35–36, 40–41, 44, 114–15, 129

identity, 11, 26, 58, 97, 99; Belizean, 35n4, 52; collective, 43, 101; construction of, 22n28; cultural, 17, 58, 60n54, 112, 119; ethnic, 23, 23n29; Garifuna, 53, 57, 60, 66, 71, 97n2, 112; group, 14; and health, 17n19, 24, 34, 43n13, 103, 126; and heritage practices, 11, 15, 62, 101; Indigenous, 56; Maya, 9, 32, 36, 38, 62, 71, 89, 89n20, 119; and taste, 35; and West Africa, 57
Indigenous communities, 58, 97, 113, 115n2, 125, 127, 137; Arawak, 22n28; Carib, 22n28; and "change", 12, 33; and disenfranchisement, 118; and economic

change, 21; and environmental change, 14, 21; and experiences, 26; and food, 60; and government policy, 38; and healers, 81; and health, 56, 120; and knowledge, 18n21, 45n14, 61n11, 91, 119, 120n6, 127; and land, 118; and leaders, 53; and mistreatment, 38, 96, 117; and Mopan, 23; and plant medicines, 81; and practices, 23, 57, 64, 83, 120; and pride, 96; and Q'echi' Maya, 23; and research, 5, 45, 80n11; and Santa Cruz, 39; and values, 106, 131; and villages, 96

knowledge, 35, 73, 87, 95–96, 103, 109, 133; ancestral, 102, 121; colonial, 128n22; cultural, 99; ecological, 17–18, 31; environmental, 17, 26; ethnobotanical, 84; and farming, 77; and health, 112; heritage, 101; Indigenous, 18n21, 45n14, 91, 119–20; and land management, 39; medicinal, 81; plant, 54, 121; and practice, 118; production of, 15; traditional, 53, 100, 130

land, 9, 20, 43, 51, 57, 63, 65, 109, 120; customary, 20; Indigenous, 39, 118; management, 38–39, 74, 119; and natural resources, 118; ownership, 21; rights, 22, 37–38, 50, 81, 84, 119, 132; tenure, 22, 31, 31n2, 37n6; traditional, 40; use, 9; village, 21, 37n6; and water, 50
language, 15, 51n1, 66n14, 71, 73, 78, 83, 90, 96, 98, 131; biocultural, 99; loss, 132, 136; medicine, 110; preservation of, 62–63
Los Angeles, 51, 93–97, 100–102, 104, 110–11, 115
Lovell, James, 98–99

Maya: and achiote, 107; and agriculture, 78; and ancestry, 31; Belizean, 23, 29, 36, 50, 90n22, 95, 106, 116; and caldo, 126; collective, 34; community, 3–5, 9, 12, 13n13, 21, 22n28, 26, 39, 43, 45, 51, 67, 81, 118–20, 131; and daily life, 7; and dance, 136; and economic model, 38; and environment, 24; and farmers, 9, 11, 74, 75n4, 77; and food, 29, 35; and health, 23, 42, 81–82, 113, 121, 127; and heritage, 33, 40, 119; and hospitality, 70, 91; and identity, 9, 32, 62n12, 69, 71, 89; and knowledge, 133; and land rights, 22, 38, 132; and land tenure, 37n6; and leaders, 79–80, 105; and livelihoods, 22; and medicine, 53, 93; and Mopan Mayans, 6, 31, 64, 100; and practices, 128; and Q'eqchi' Mayans, 64, 130; and Toledo, 124; and traditions, 40, 61–62, 70, 77–78; and values, 32, 36, 41, 79, 85–86, 92, 106; and villages, 14, 20, 31n2, 37n7, 49–50, 84, 86; and women, 104
medical care, 83, 115
medical personnel, 41
medical science, 61n11
medicine, 40–41, 53, 93, 121; and biomedicine, 52, 82–83, 117, 129; ethnobotanical, 91; herbal, 14, 24, 54; and plants, 23, 70n1, 81–82, 90–91, 101, 133–34; and practices, 52, 81; and teas, 52; traditional, 99n4, 110, 133
money, 9, 38, 46–47, 67, 79, 83, 92, 109, 113; and biomedical system, 24; and education, 33, 35, 73; and subsistence, 20, 29
music: Garifuna, 66, 99–100; marimba, 86; percussive, 135; and sensory practice, 87n19, 132;

traditional, 18, 24, 42, 62, 86–87, 92, 112

nature, 18n21, 80, 89–90, 124–25

plants, 33, 42, 55, 66, 74, 84, 94, 120, 122, 134; and Belize, 53; cacao, 73; and cultivation, 64, 74, 77, 79–80, 85; and healing chemicals, 121; and knowledge, 121; local, 6, 65, 132; and Maya peoples, 32; medicinal, 23, 70n1, 81–82, 83, 90–91, 101, 133–34; and relationships, 65; and spirituality, 121; traditional, 15, 54, 99; wild, 18
Punta Gorda, 50, 64, 80, 83, 108, 114, 118, 121, 131

reciprocal labor, 31–32, 79
reciprocal practice, 64

Santa Cruz, 6, 14, 16, 19–20, 27, 46, 49–51, 61, 67, 114–15, 136; and bush medicine, 83; and caldo, 71; and Caye Caulker, 33n3; and community centers, 128; and Deer Dance, 85, 92, 135; and farming, 73–74; and food, 34–35; and Garifuna language, 62; and health, 40; and identity, 44; and Jose Mes, 69; and k'uxub, 104; and land ownership, 21; and Maya people, 39, 84; and Mopan Maya, 31; and music, 86–87; and parents, 28; and Southern Highway, 86; and technology, 75; and traditions, 86; and women, 130
science, 60n11, 61n11, 73, 75–76, 103, 117, 127, 137
sensory engagement, 24
sensory ethnography, 7

sensory experience, 7, 15, 17, 26, 43n13, 60, 71, 82, 99, 101, 117, 122, 125, 127, 129, 131, 133, 135
sensory nostalgia, 121, 122n7
sensory pathways, 77
sensory practice, 87n19
sensory therapeutics, 126
social action, 82n15
social conditions, 13n14, 14, 79, 124–25; and biology, 71; and environment, 74; and DNA, 58; and indigeneity, 40; and physical conditions, 15
social isolation, 132
social justice, 99
social knowledge, 26
social life, 102
social marginalization, 22
social media, 64, 84–85, 108, 111–12, 132
social organization, 9–10
social relations, 41, 131
social structures, 11, 120
space, 5, 25, 43, 55, 60, 63–65, 118, 121–22, 134, 137n31

time, 5, 25, 43, 55, 60, 64, 118, 122
Toledo, 4, 24, 31, 37n6, 42, 72, 105–6, 118, 121, 124
Toledo Alcaldes Association (TAA), 37n7, 38, 64, 77n9, 79
tradition, 25, 33, 47, 79–80, 96, 101, 104n7, 111, 123, 130–31, 134; and capitalism, 119; and commodification, 119; and communities, 17, 38; and dance, 18, 86, 135n30; and ecological practices, 14, 16, 19n25, 31, 42, 73; and farming practices, 9, 20–21, 74, 77–78, 132; and foods, 15–16, 18, 34, 58, 69–70, 107, 110, 112, 124; Garifuna, 4, 63, 107;

and governance, 37; and healing, 83–84, 90, 117, 127, 131; heritage, 21, 96; and housing, 32; and land management, 38–40; language, 63; and learning practices, 90; and livelihoods, 37; loss of, 14; maintaining, 57, 76, 130n24; and Maya values, 36, 40–41, 67, 70, 77, 85; and medicinal practices, 52, 63, 81–82, 99n4, 110, 133; and music, 24, 42, 62, 66, 86–87, 92; and plants, 15, 54, 81, 83–84, 99, 121; and practices, 6, 17, 41, 53, 57, 61–63, 84–86, 91, 102–3, 112, 116–18, 120, 124, 128–29, 132, 136–37; and resources, 22; and rights, 21; and rituals, 43; and stories, 66; West African, 57
traditional ecological knowledge (TEK), 17–18, 31
traditional ecological practices, 14, 16, 19n25, 42, 73

United Nations Declaration on the Rights of Indigenous Peoples (UNDRIP), 20
United Nations Permanent Forum on Indigenous Issues, 37
United States, 6, 8n4, 10, 16, 24, 52, 58, 65, 78, 100, 104, 109, 118; and Belize, 80, 95; and city, 135; and cultural identity, 60n10; and diasporas, 51, 98, 103, 105, 107–8; and food, 35, 111n11; and migration, 56, 107; and migrant health, 18, 130; and public health, 102; and tourism, 96
universities, 67, 73, 84, 92

villages, 3, 34–35, 46–47, 77, 87, 97, 118; and Caye Caulker, 33, 69; and dances, 92; and Dangriga, 67; and development projects, 128; and education, 28; and elders, 75, 124; and farms, 31–32, 44, 75; fishing, 49, 102; and food, 109; and governance, 79; and health clinic, 83; and Hopkins, 50; Indigenous, 96; and land, 21, 37n6, 50; and leadership positions, 69, 85; Maya, 49, 69, 84, 89; and Maya values, 36; and membership, 79; and men, 31–32; Mopan Maya, 14; Placencia, 103; and plants, 91; and police, 50; and Q'eqchi', 105; and Santa Cruz, 19–20, 31, 33, 42, 73, 86, 114–15; and Seine Bight, 110; and Uxbenká, 39; and women, 20–21

wellness, 5n1, 11, 17–18, 23, 54, 62, 64, 71, 76, 89, 132

ABOUT THE AUTHOR

Kristina Baines is a sociocultural anthropologist with an applied medical/environmental focus. Her research interests include Indigenous ecologies, health, and heritage in the context of global change, in addition to publicly engaged research and dissemination practices. She is professor of anthropology at the City University of New York, Guttman Community College, affiliated faculty at the CUNY Graduate School of Public Health and Health Policy, and director of anthropology for *Cool Anthropology*. Her co-edited book of the same name was released in 2022. Her first book, *Embodying Ecological Heritage in Maya Community: Health, Happiness, and Identity*, was published in 2016.